PICTURES OF HEALTH

A PHOTOGRAPHIC HISTORY OF HEALTH CARE IN PHILADELPHIA
1860–1945

JANET GOLDEN

AND

CHARLES E. ROSENBERG

UNIVERSITY OF PENNSYLVANIA PRESS · PHILADELPHIA

Library of Congress Cataloging-in-Publication Data

Golden, Janet Lynne, 1951–
    Pictures of health : a photographic history of health care in Philadelphia,
    1860–1945 / Janet Golden and Charles E. Rosenberg.
        p.   cm.
    Includes bibliographical references and index.
    ISBN 0-8122-8237-X (cloth). — ISBN 0-8122-1311-4 (pbk.)
    1. Medical care—Pennsylvania—Philadelphia—History.   2. Medical care—
Pennsylvania—Philadelphia—History—Pictorial works.   2. Medicine—Penn-
sylvania—Philadelphia—History—Pictorial works.   I. Rosenberg, Charles E.
II. Title.
RA395.A4P43   1991
362.1′09748′11—dc20   90-22745
                                                                        CIP

Contents

List of Photographs

IN WRITING A photographic history of health care in Philadelphia we have learned much about the city and about health care. We have been able to see in images what we had before "seen" only in words. We have also had the difficult task of selecting a sample from among the literally thousands of photographs that collectively tell the story of how Philadelphians received and delivered health services in the years before 1945. We could not simply cull the less informative pictures, nor could we choose only the most visually arresting. We sought instead to illustrate the several themes that are the focus of this book: the education and training of health professionals, the delivery of care in hospitals, the work of care givers, and the efforts to improve and protect the public's health.

While the book uses an expansive definition of health, and includes pictures ranging from the city's "Rat Patrol" to a late-nineteenth-century anatomy lecture at the University of Pennsylvania, several kinds of images have been omitted. There are no formal portraits of the many great and famous physicians and nurses who studied and practiced in Philadelphia. Nor are there any images illustrating the ways in which photography has contributed to the study of medicine, although this too is a subject with Philadelphia roots. From the famous "walking man" images of Eadweard Muybridge to the pictures used for recording a variety of clinical syndromes, photography and its kindred arts such as medical illustration have played a vital role in medicine. Finally, we have excluded pictures of the many women and men who went abroad from Philadelphia to staff base hospitals or otherwise served in the military, who worked as medical missionaries around the world, or who after study in Philadelphia made important contributions elsewhere. These individuals helped Philadelphia to earn its designation as a medical center for the world, but their stories are better told elsewhere.

Almost all the photographs in this collection were taken between 1890 and 1945. While there are early photographs of health care in Philadelphia, particularly of the city's Civil War hospitals, it was not until the late nineteenth century that photographs began to be taken of the varied health care activities within the city. This was a reflection more of the technical complexity of photography than of a lack of skill or curiosity among the city's photographers. After 1945 the opposite problem occurs. There are too many images and they are too skillfully produced. The abundance of public relations materials—the smiling patients, the tidy hospital rooms, the dramatic images of surgeons, and the pictures of sick young children—as well as other stylized and carefully staged photographs, are too numerous and too familiar. While it would be inviting to include these images, make com-

Preface

parisons, and see medicine "then and now," with its singular advances and its growing complexity, we have instead chosen to focus on the "then." We want to tell a story of Philadelphia health care that is unfamiliar, even as it reveals the roots of many of our contemporary practices and institutions.

Perhaps a word is in order about the creation of this book. Both authors worked on the organizational scheme; Janet Golden selected the pictures and wrote the first draft of the text, and Charles Rosenberg wrote the introduction. The final draft was a collaboration.

MANY ARCHIVISTS AND librarians and others made this book possible, helping us to find, interpret, and reproduce the photographs included in *Pictures of Health*. We would like to thank Stanley Arnold, Afro-American Historical and Cultural Museum; Robert Eskind, Atwater Kent Museum; Patricia Proscino, Balch Institute for Ethnic Studies; Shirley Bonnem, Children's Hospital of Philadelphia; Thomas Horrocks, Jean Carr, and Jack Eckert, Historical Collections of the College of Physicians of Philadelphia; Barbara Williams, Hahnemann University Archives and History of Medicine Collection; Marcy Silver, Historical Society of Philadelphia; Kenneth Finkel, Library Company of Philadelphia; Jill Gates Smith, Archives and Special Collections on Women in Medicine of the Medical College of Pennsylvania; Caroline Morris, Archives of the Pennsylvania Hospital; Lee Stanley, Philadelphia City Archives; Charles Blockson and Richard Beards, Blockson Collection, Temple University; Carol Ann Harris, Conwellana-Templana Collection of Temple University; George Brightbill, Pamela Austin, and Brenda Galloway, Urban Archives, Temple University; Judith Robbins, Thomas Jefferson University Archives; Mark Lloyd and Sandra Markham, University of Pennsylvania Archives; David Weinberg, Center for the History of the Study of Nursing, University of Pennsylvania; Linda Walsh, School of Nursing of the University of Pennsylvania; and I. Maximillian Martin.

We also wish to thank Julie Johnson for assistance with research and the bibliography; Rick Echelmeyer, who took a number of the photographs; and those individuals who commented on various portions of the manuscript: Barbara Bates, Joel Howell, Nancy Tomes, and Eric Schneider.

This book is dedicated to our families: Eric Schneider, Alexander Schneider, and Benjamin Schneider; Drew Faust, Leah Rosenberg, and Jessica Rosenberg.

Acknowledgments

REPRESENTING MEDICINE: PHILADELPHIA, HEALTH, AND
PHOTOGRAPHY, 1860–1945   *Charles E. Rosenberg*

THE YEAR 1989 MARKED THE 150th anniversary of photography. During that
century and a half, the camera, medicine, and urban society have participated
in a complex and multidimensional relationship. The following pages seek
to illuminate the contours of that relationship, to show how the camera was
used to represent the world of medicine in one American city, Philadelphia.

Represented, not mirrored. For photography provides not a necessarily
balanced and self-evident picture of medical care and medicine, but one of
certain portions of that world, recorded not by relatively disinterested social
historians or archivists, but by men—and some women—involved in institutional medicine. They were individuals with a story to tell and a limited
yet fascinating new medium in which to tell it.

Ante-bellum Philadelphia was a leader in medical education and publishing as well as in applied science and technology. The Quaker City's active
and alert technical community experimented with the daguerreotype process
within weeks after the first descriptions were published in Paris in August
1839.[1] And just as modern photography has evolved into a genre that would
hardly have been recognized by its inquisitive mid-nineteenth-century practitioners, so medicine has grown into a complex of ideas, institutions, and
practices that would not be easily grasped by nineteenth-century clinicians.
Only the fundamental social basis of medicine remains unaltered: the reality
of perceived illness or injury and the consequent need to provide care.

Introduction

Philadelphia Medicine, 1870–1945:
An Era of Change

Medical education, its repertoire of ideas, tools, techniques, and patterns of
clinical practice, and the profession's institutional and economic bases have
all undergone profound changes during the past century; even the incidence
of sickness has shifted dramatically. And much of this change took place
during the pivotal half-century following 1875.

The limits built into the human body have hardly changed, however. For
those fit enough to survive the hazards of infancy and childhood, life expectancies in the mid-nineteenth century were not radically different from those
prevalent in the United States today. But many did not survive those early
years. Life expectancy was roughly 40 for Americans in 1880—half of what
it is today. For big-city dwellers, it could be much lower. In Philadelphia
in 1880, life expectancy at birth was 40.2 for white males and 44.8 for
white females, and 25.2 and 32.1 respectively for black males and females.

A forty-year-old Philadelphian might live to 65 if a man and almost 69 if a women; for blacks the figures were 58.6 and 64.[2] Although a smaller proportion of Americans survived to die of the degenerative diseases now preeminent in tables of mortality, their experience with them (except for an apparently much lower incidence of most kinds of cancer) was similar to those of the late twentieth century.[3]

On the other hand, infant mortality—which provides an excellent index to general living conditions—remained dismayingly high in the 1880s, far closer to the figures for late-twentieth-century Bangladesh or Chad.[4] In 1870, almost one of five Philadelphia infants died before reaching its first birthday; another 15 percent died by their fifth birthday.[5] Infectious disease was still a key element in those deaths; infant diarrhoeas, fevers, and pneumonias were the major killers. By 1930 the situation was very different—and very much closer to late-twentieth-century realities. Seventy-five of a thousand infants died before their first birthday and twenty-three before attaining their fifth year—a dramatic improvement over the situation a half-century earlier. And these changes took place before the advent of antibiotics or modern techniques for dealing with the dehydration, pneumonias, and other age-old killers of infants and young children.

Many sorts of change were taking place simultaneously in late-nineteenth-century Philadelphia, with developments in medicine and health intricately linked to every aspect of material and institutional change. It is hard, indeed, to draw a firm boundary between the medical and non-medical in their impact on the incidence of disease and life expectancy. Improvements in diet, for example, had an important effect on both morbidity and mortality in the late nineteenth century, when a revolution in the transportation and preservation of foodstuffs and in the economic organization and technical underpinnings of agriculture had made an increasing variety of foods available to urban working people for an ever-smaller percentage of their income. Cheaper soap and clothing had a parallel effect, as did a gradual improvement in the quality of housing.[6] Access to more abundant and less contaminated water supplies and effective sewage systems also helped reduce the chances of sickness and premature death. Such amenities implied not only laboratory knowledge but the practical skills of civil engineers, business people, and politicians. All these factors interacted to produce better living conditions for ordinary Philadelphians—and thus a more disease-resistant and longer-lived population.

Modern historians agree with contemporaries in finding the mid-nineteenth-century city a dangerous place, inimical to the men and women who moved there from farms and villages seeking work in the burgeoning metropolitan economies. Pioneer nineteenth-century students of mortality patterns were unanimous in concluding that urban death rates were appreciably higher and life expectancies lower than were their rural counterparts.

Philadelphia was in most respects typical of this pattern. America's largest city at the time of independence, it continued to increase steadily in absolute size and population as it attracted in-migrants from rural America and Europe—first from the British Isles and Germany, then by the end of the century from Southern and Eastern Europe. These new Philadelphians provided labor for the city's industries and transportation network; they lived in crowded and unhealthy tenement districts and died in disproportionate numbers from tuberculosis and typhoid, as their children did from "summer diarrhoea" and other infectious ills.

Although it had fallen well behind New York in numbers and economic significance by mid-century, the Quaker City continued to be a center of medical teaching, practice, publishing, and writing. And while Philadelphia medicine continued to provide national leadership, medicine itself changed dramatically in the three quarters of a century before 1940.

Many of the key developments were technical: medical care had become increasingly identified with laboratories and machines. By 1900, innovations such as the x-ray, antiseptic surgery, and preventive immunizations had become central to medicine's public image and future promise. Urban health care was already specialized and was often delivered in institutional settings, not in physicians' offices or middle-class homes as it had been in the last quarter of the nineteenth century. Much nineteenth-century medical care was, in fact, not provided by full-time credentialed physicians at all; family, friends, neighbors, and druggists provided first lines of clinical defense in their several ways. By 1925, however, hospital beds and outpatient examining rooms had become crucial to the delivery of care to urban Americans of every social class, not simply to the dependent, as had still been the case in 1875. By 1925 as well, physicians, like members of other professions and many skilled occupations, were being uniformly educated, systematically licensed, and increasingly autonomous within a largely self-regulating organizational structure.

Many aspects of this new medicine were related organically to urban growth. The scale of illness, for example, encouraged the development of hospital facilities; the availability of hospital facilities implied the need for house staff and the possibility of clinical training. Medical schools sought gradually to integrate these clinical opportunities into their curricula. The growth of specialties too was integrated closely with the concentration of population in urban areas: the referral fees of the wealthy permitted an economically viable specialized practice while the sick poor filled hospital beds and outpatient consulting rooms and provided opportunities for clinical instruction.[7] The growth of public welfare, institutional health care, and medical education were all symbiotically intertwined—all aspects of the multifaceted evolution of urban life. Similarly, public health programs developed in response to an increasing burden of illness and the perception that urban filth and crowding could no longer be tolerated; disease had to be prevented as well as treated.[8]

The intellectual world of medicine also provided new tools for understanding and averting infectious disease. The germ theory was the most conspicuous of such tools and the most significant in its implications for preventive medicine. Medical opinion had long agreed that the great majority of those ills peculiarly associated with urban poor health, with endemic infant mortality and recurrent epidemics, were "unnecessary" and avoidable. The very differences between rural and urban life expectancies provided a powerful argument for eradicating those ills that shortened the lives of city dwellers. Most of the ailments that accounted for the excess in urban over rural mortality were classified by mid-nineteenth-century authorities as zymotic (from their linguistic and metaphoric root in the process of fermentation) or infectious ills. But the mechanism accounting for the spread of such ills remained obscure until the generation of Pasteur and Koch. The germ theory of disease and wound infection, which gradually found acceptance in the world's medical community between the mid-1860s and the 1880s, seemed to provide an explanation for the infectiousness of many ills—and imply a set of strategies for preventing them.

Thus the end of the nineteenth and early years of the twentieth century were the heroic age of public health, of the attempt to change the living conditions and life-styles of urban dwellers so that they might live longer and less illness-marred lives; of efforts to interdict the spread of pathogenic microorganisms by diagnosis, isolation, and quarantine; of a commitment to develop and enforce preventive immunizations. All these new public health goals—improved sewerage and environmental sanitation, the application of bacteriology, health education, the campaign against tuberculosis and infant mortality, as well as improved hospital and home care—can be traced to this dynamic period in the history of medicine. And all were recorded in photography, a medium that embodied and symbolized the novel technologies that seemed to be transforming America's urban world.

The Photographer and the Medical System

Historians of medicine overlap in many ways with historians generally; one of them is in an habitual privileging of the written word. Artifacts and images remain marginal to the work of most professional historians. This lack of concern is particularly egregious in the modern period, when photography has played so prominent a role in recording, rationalizing, and communicating medicine's collective image and—in clinical and microscopical contexts—constituting an aspect of medicine's intellectual as well as social identity.[9]

This latter aspect of medical photography will not be covered in the following pages. We do not reproduce photographs taken with the intent of representing clinical entities. We do not reproduce, to cite another sort of example, the celebrated—and Philadelphia-based—experiments of Eadweard Muybridge in using the camera to understand the mechanism of animal locomotion. More generally significant was the use of the camera to record the microscope's insights—and we do not reproduce examples of nineteenth-century photomicrographs. These technical uses of the camera represent elusive problems of intellectual context, of disciplinary convention and authorial intent, questions that demand specialized analysis. The following pages will deal largely with medicine's social aspect, with the presentation of its institutions, practices, and personnel to itself and to a larger world. Collectively such images constituted part of the multidimensional interface connecting the medical community with society generally.

As we are well aware, and despite their invocation of time-distanced authenticity, photographs are not simply candid slices of past life recorded by a necessarily neutral and unreflective lens; each image presents a stylized and highly crafted arrangement of reality. We must read these pictures as the artfully composed texts they are—reflecting both unexamined cultural assumptions and conscious institutional needs. The photographs that follow represent images of real rooms, real people, real practices, but in unique configurations incorporating ideological assumption, institutional interest, cultural and aesthetic convention, and technical constraint. We should not see this mode of constructing images as coming between us and a "truth" the unreflective lens and shutter might otherwise have recorded, but as a valuable clue to the equally real world of interest and ideology that interacted to configure particular surviving photographs.

The historian seeking to use photographs to help understand the world in which they were made is limited in some ways by the accidents of time, circumstance, and shifting value that have determined not only whether and in which circumstances a picture was taken but whether it would be preserved—and if preserved whether it would be in an accessible institutional collection. This book is thus inevitably not a well-balanced picture of medical care as it was in fact experienced by past actors, but a view of a narrow sector of that care, in particular the institutional—the medical school and hospital, the dispensary, the visiting nurse service, and an assortment of municipal health programs.

The private practice of medicine, on the other hand, is not adequately recorded in photographs. One reason, of course, lies in conventions of modesty and privacy; not surprisingly we have no photographic records of nurses emptying bedpans, let alone patients using them, nor do we have photographs of ordinary patients sick in their homes, or being treated by family physicians. Class too determined the form and content of photographs; almost all patients depicted by late-nineteenth- and early-twentieth-century photographers were "charity" patients in institutional settings. And the institution's needs and self-perceptions had much to do with the content of such images. Middle-class patients were as little likely to be photographed in their private or semi-private rooms as they were in their homes. The taking of a photograph was a kind of ritual and implied an appropriately meaningful occasion and subject matter. Medical photographs were in their early years largely celebratory (when they were not efforts at clinical documentation), recordings of the special and memorable, not the routine and "uninteresting," and certainly not the "indecent" or intrusive.

Photography, as we are all aware, is distinguished by its ambiguous epistemological and perceptual status. The seeming "objectivity" of the photograph as artifact lulls most viewers into the casual assumption that photographic images are somehow a candid and unambiguous, unconstructed, version of reality. Composed of elements seemingly concrete and unambiguous (and resonant with the alienness of past experience), they project an insidious pseudo-veracity. At the same time, the photograph is inevitably construed by individuals viewing it as a moment in a narrative that precedes and inevitably continues beyond the moment the shutter opened. The viewer is thus obligate storyteller and hermeneuticist, imposing meaning and structure on a particular image.

But the stories tend to be archetypical, representing structured social relationships as much as the particular stories in which these relationships are acted out. The medical images we reproduce are thus collectively a kind of *tableau vivant,* representing and thus legitimating existing social hierarchies and roles. Let me refer, by way of example, to the stylized image of the turn-of-the-century visiting nurse in her client's tenement apartment, the nurse with her status-embodying hat and carefully ironed shirtwaist, the patient grateful, neat, and passive. Both protagonists are acting out assumed and contrasting roles, consciously posed and presumably reassuring to the agency's middle- and upper-class supporters.

The photographs in this volume were taken largely by anonymous men and women and represent a kind of collective vernacular style. Nevertheless, most photographs taken in hospitals or public health programs were clearly "official," meant to represent a considered institutional vision. The numerous hospital photographs of the period illustrate this nicely. They capture and project a vision of order, cleanliness, grateful patients, well-scrubbed wards, tastefully decorated private rooms, and carefully groomed nurses. These images of order and hierarchy in status, profession, and gender were certainly intended to reassure donors and prospective private patients. Thus, only in images of Philadelphia General, a municipal hospital that boasted neither, do we glimpse something of the often disorderly reality that constituted late-nineteenth-century institutional care. Slow shutter speeds and film reinforce the assumption of static roles and rigid hierarchies. Individuals stand at rigid attention, acting out formal places in a social hierarchy.

Reassuring in a different—but ultimately consistent—way was an emphasis on the hospital's growing technical capacity. The camera was quick to record gleaming surgical amphitheaters, apparatus for rehabilitation, and diagnostic laboratories. The surgical amphitheater or operating room constituted a particularly important and often photographed setting; for it provided an arena in which could be acted out not only the promise of technology but the continuing status of the physician-operator as individual—of the surgical intervention as battle-piece with the surgeon as protagonist/champion in the struggle against death and incapacity. Like the public health nurse's tenement visit, the operation was one of the ritual genre scenes framed again and again by photographers of medicine.[10]

Policy, ideology, and aesthetics all interacted to produce such conventional emphases and images. Children, for example, are far more prominent in these medical images than men and women at the end of life. Children represent the potential for social activism and the urgent need for imposing order as well as health; boys and girls depicted on hospital wards, in school-rooms, or in dispensaries were products of the city's tenements, embodying both the promise and menace for the next generation. American social welfare has demonstrated a long-standing preference for work with children, and Progressive-era photographers carried this policy emphasis forward, well aware of the appeal implicit in the children's expressive eyes and vulnerable bodies. Sentimentality and calculation interacted to produce countless images of children whose minds and bodies demanded salvation.

Many of the images in public health are—like those of children in such contexts—self-consciously staged exercises in public relations. Nevertheless they tell us which elements seemed most compelling and plausible to contemporaries. In reading these pictures we must keep all of these factors in mind—aesthetic convention and institutional interest, technical limitation, and cultural assumption—even the simple desire to record images of one's friends, oneself, one's colleagues. The ultimate elusiveness of their seemingly transparent reality only adds to the hold these historic images exert over their viewer's imagination. They provide an indispensable access to an exotic yet somehow familiar past.

Notes

1. A daguerreotype image of Central High School made in all probability at the end of September 1839 is a strong claimant to being the oldest surviving North American photograph. Cf. William F. Stapp, *Robert Cornelius: Portraits from the Dawn of Photography* (Washington, D.C.: Smithsonian Institution Press for the National Portrait Gallery, 1983), pp. 27–28, 41, 47.

2. For more detailed accounts of medical care in this period, see Charles E. Rosenberg, "Between Two Worlds: American Medicine in 1879," in John Blake, ed., *Centenary of Index Medicus* (Washington, D.C.: U.S. Government Printing Office, 1980), pp. 3–18; "What It Was Like to Be Sick in 1884," *American Heritage* 35 (1984): 22–31.

3. In 1980, Philadelphia's death rate was 1,247.6 per 100,000; the leading individual causes were heart, 413.5 and malignant neoplasms, 263.7. Philadelphia Department of Public Health, *Annual Statistical Report, 1980. Division of Health Program Analysis* (Philadelphia: City of Philadelphia, n.d.), p. 22.

4. In certain portions of the American community, death rates after five have remained inordinately high. A 1990 study in the *New England Journal of Medicine,* for example, reports that African American males in New York's Harlem have a life expectancy shorter than their counterparts in Bangladesh. Colin McCord and Harold

Freeman, "Excess Mortality in Harlem," *New England Journal of Medicine* 322 (Jan. 18, 1990): 173–177.

5. Gretchen A. Condran and Rose A. Cheney, "Mortality Trends in Philadelphia: Age- and Cause-Specific Death Rates, 1870–1930," *Demography* 19 (1982): 100.

6. Tuberculosis incidence constitutes a particularly sensitive indicator of response to such multifaceted environmental variables. And contemporaries were aware that the tuberculosis rate had begun to decline in the nineteenth century before there was any effective therapeutic intervention available. Thomas McKeown has in recent years used such material to underline the need for concern with social factors and to question the tendency to grant too much credit to specific medical interventions in the demographic transition. See Thomas McKeown, *The Role of Medicine: Dream, Mirage, or Nemesis?* (Princeton, N.J.: Princeton University Press, 1979); Gillian Cronje, "Tuberculosis and Mortality Decline in England and Wales, 1851–1900," in Robert Wood and John Woodward, eds., *Urban Disease and Mortality in Nineteenth-Century England* (London and New York: St. Martin's Press, 1984), pp. 79–101.

7. For a more detailed analysis of hospital development, see Charles E. Rosenberg, *The Care of Strangers: The Rise of America's Hospital System* (New York: Basic Books, 1987); Rosemary Stevens, *In Sickness and in Wealth: American Hospitals in the Twentieth Century* (New York: Basic Books, 1989). There is no recent synthetic study of Philadelphia hospitals. On the medical profession and its relationship to hospitals, however, see Leo J. O'Hara, *An Emerging Profession: Philadelphia Doctors, 1860–1900* (New York: Garland, 1989).

8. For a general account, see Edward T. Morman, "Scientific Medicine Comes to Philadelphia: Public Health Transformed, 1854–1899," unpub. Ph.D. dissertation, University of Pennsylvania, 1986.

9. For a recent attempt to contextualize medical photographs in this period, see Daniel M. Fox and Christopher Lawrence, *Photographing Medicine: Images and Power in Britain and America Since 1840* (Westport, Conn. and London: Greenwood, 1988).

10. Many of the these surgical photographs were in fact posed, with medical students or house officers impersonating the patient.

PICTURES OF HEALTH

ONE

Training for the New Professions

BETWEEN 1880 AND 1945 medical education and nursing education underwent significant changes. The hospital, the site of formal nursing education since its inception, also became the locus of medical training for all physicians and not just a small minority of the ambitious and well connected.

By the early twentieth century the standard medical school curriculum began to encompass laboratory work and small-group bedside instruction as well as didactic lectures. In the mid-nineteenth century only the medical elite completed their training in a hospital; by the 1920s every new practitioner gained experience in its wards and operating rooms. Formal residency programs were now available for would-be specialists, internship was required of all, and many of Philadelphia's hospitals had become educational as well as healing institutions.

Unlike medical education, nursing education had always taken place in the hospital wards. On-the-job training had prepared thousands of women for professional service since the opening of America's first nursing schools in the early 1870s. What changed, in the period covered by the photographs we have reproduced here, was both the scientific and technical complexity of the hospital and the amount of time devoted to classroom training. Nursing leaders labored to redefine the relationship between nursing education as intellectual training and as task-oriented apprenticeship by limiting the hours spent in practical work and increasing the time devoted to the study of nursing theory. Internal reforms within nursing schools coupled with the hospital's growing reliance upon a work force composed of trained nurses rather than nursing students led to a reshaping of nursing education in the last two-thirds of the twentieth century. Today, nursing education begins in the college classroom.

The photographs document the physical settings in which professional training took place, showing medical students in school lecture halls and laboratories, as well as in hospital wards, clinics, and operating rooms. Similarly, nurses are shown at the bedside and in the classroom. But the images communicate more than the everyday experiences of these young students and trainees. They display their attempts to represent themselves as proud members of scientific professions. The uniforms they wear—nurses in hospital school caps; residents in suits, or in the case of those serving at the Philadelphia General Hospital, military-style coats—convey their status. Similarly, by choosing ambulances as the backdrop for their group portraits, these aspiring professionals show that they see themselves as participating in the expanding world of hospital medicine. Thus the photographs, like education itself, transmit both a slice of visible past life and something rather less tangible, a generation's self-image.

AMERICA'S FIRST MEDICAL school, what was then the College of Philadelphia and is now the University of Pennsylvania School of Medicine, opened its doors in 1765. At a time when the great majority of American practitioners acquired their education through apprenticeship, the creation of a formal institution of learning constituted a bold step.

During the first half of the nineteenth century apprenticeship remained the most common route to a medical career, although the popularity and number of medical schools was growing. Most were simply profit-making institutions offering short lecture courses open to anyone who paid a fee; little regard was paid to prior education or attainment, although it was assumed that matriculants would have served a period of apprenticeship before (or during) their medical school days. With no meaningfully enforced licensing requirements to impede them, the graduates of these medical schools could begin practicing medicine without having been trained in bedside care, in some cases without ever having laid eyes and hands upon a patient. Only a minority could attend one of the better schools such as Pennsylvania, Jefferson, or Harvard; even fewer supplemented their education with further study in Europe or served as house officers in one of the nation's few hospitals. From the elite group who enjoyed these opportunities came the leaders who were to advocate reforms in medical education during the late nineteenth and early twentieth centuries.

Reform had four components: establishing licensing requirements for practitioners, weeding out weak medical schools, raising admission standards for those seeking medical careers, and strengthening the scientific and clinical training of those attending the better schools. In Philadelphia these changes were felt in numerous ways. The state enacted a licensing law in 1875, which was amended in 1877 to require a diploma from a medical college, with an exemption for those in practice for five years. By 1893, with schools of doubtful quality still flourishing, the state established three medical boards, one for regular physicians, one for homeopathic physicians, and one for eclectic physicians. These boards attempted to set educational standards by denying certification to applicants with diplomas from unaccredited schools. The state established a three-year curriculum, which was extended to four years in 1911. The toughened licensing requirements—paralleling policies enacted in a good many other states—drove many of the diploma mills out of business.

Standards were raised in the surviving institutions. Students entering the University of Pennsylvania School of Medicine in 1908, for example, were required to have attended one year of college, and the following year admission required two years of college work. Instead of a four-month course of lectures, repeated a second time the following year, students studied for three and eventually four years. The first two years typically combined didactic lectures with practical science courses. The last two years emphasized clinical observation; all matriculants now learned medicine by cutting, probing, touching, and experimenting as well as by listening.

The changing pattern at the University of Pennsylvania was paralleled among its competitors. Hahnemann Medical College and Hospital offered a three-year graded curriculum in 1869, which became mandatory in 1886. In 1890 it began offering a four-year curriculum, which became mandatory in 1894. Students at Hahnemann still studied the therapeutic and etiological principles elaborated by the German physician Samuel Hahnemann (1775–1843). Known as homeopathy, this system emphasized the use of highly diluted doses of drugs that were believed to have a dynamic effect on the body. Homeopathic physicians not only challenged the beliefs of orthodox practitioners, but also created an alternative system of medical education and hospital care. During the late nineteenth century homeopathic and orthodox physicians gradually began to converge in terms of doctrine and to compromise in terms of professional relations. By the First World War, Hahnemann students pursued a curriculum that in most respects was similar to those required by their peers at Pennsylvania, Jefferson, Temple, and the Woman's Medical College (since 1970 the Medical College of Pennsylvania).

The most significant development in medical education in the twentieth century occurred when hospital internships became a standard part of medical training for all students, not just an opportunity to be enjoyed by a minority. The medical education that began in the classroom and laboratory concluded in hospital wards and operating rooms, a transformation that changed the meaning of hospital care, as well as medical training.

Advances in photographic technology coincided with the transformation of medical education, allowing us to see into the dissection rooms and laboratories that developed at the end of the nineteenth century. Though primitive in appearance by late-twentieth-century standards, these facilities heralded the gradual emergence of scientific medicine and of practitioners able to apply newly discovered scientific principles. Perhaps the most striking impact of this new science, visually as well as medically, occurred in the operating room, as ever more sterile conditions prevailed. It is no surprise that white-gowned surgeons in their aseptic operating theaters should have come, by the opening of the twentieth century, to symbolize medicine's new status, promise, and scientific identity. Surviving photographs record—as they once communicated—this significant new reality.

TABLE 1 Philadelphia's Medical Schools

NAME	DATE FOUNDED
University of Pennsylvania School of Medicine	1765
Thomas Jefferson University	1825
Hahnemann Medical College and Hospital	1848
Medical College of Pennsylvania	1850
Philadelphia College of Osteopathic Medicine	1898
Temple University School of Medicine	1901

1.

Leidy lecturing in pit with skulls, University of Pennsylvania School of Medicine.
University of Pennsylvania Archives.

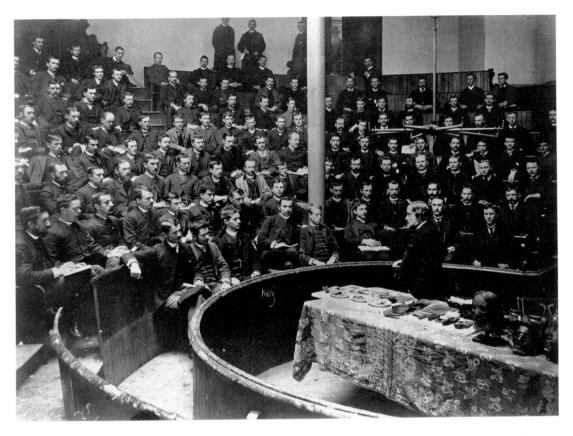

TAKEN IN 1888, this photograph shows a lecture by Dr. Joseph Leidy (1823–1891), Professor of Anatomy and director of the department of biology at the University of Pennsylvania School of Medicine. In this image Leidy, late in his career, is giving a demonstrative lecture in the "bull pit." On the table beside him are bones, skulls, and other anatomical objects.

Leidy, the foremost American anatomist of his day, held a number of positions at the university and in other institutions. His interests and skills were far-ranging: he corresponded with Charles Darwin about paleopathology, for example, and made a major contribution to medicine by discovering that trichinosis could be transmitted through uncooked pork.

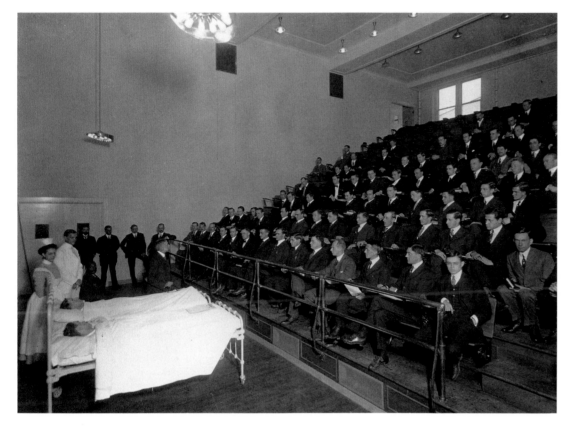

Bedridden patients in amphitheater, Gibson Wing, Hospital of the University of Pennsylvania. *University of Pennsylvania Archives.*

THIS PICTURE shows the Gibson Wing of the Hospital of the University of Pennsylvania, where women and men suffering from heart and lung diseases as well as other chronic ailments received care.

Not until the late nineteenth century, with the introduction of the clinical clerkship, would bedside teaching become a regular part of the standard medical curriculum. Prior to that time, patients were brought into the amphitheater and their condition discussed by the professor. As one student at the University of Pennsylvania recalled of his classes in the 1890s, "It really made no difference what ailed the patient; the professor could use him as text for almost any disease and we would be none the wiser." The students in this photograph, unlike most of their nineteenth-century predecessors, were able to see patients in the clinics and wards as well as in the amphitheater.

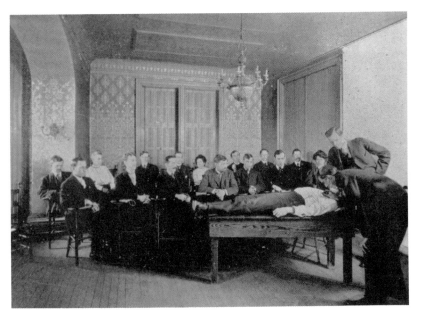

IN 1899 THE Philadelphia College and Infirmary of Osteopathy was established to teach a science of "drugless healing." Osteopathy was based on the belief that the body contained within it the elements necessary for healing and that proper manual adjustment would distribute these fluids and forces. Although it began as an irregular form of medicine, establishing its own principles, educational institutions, and hospitals, it has evolved along a path increasingly parallel to that of regular medicine in its educational standards as well as its methods of diagnosis and treatment. Nevertheless, osteopathy continues to maintain separate institutions. In the first image, students at the college are being instructed in physical diagnosis, in the second, in osteopathic diagnosis.

3.

Physical diagnosis, College of Osteopathy. *Historical Collections, College of Physicians of Philadelphia.*

4.

Osteopathic diagnosis, College of Osteopathy. *Historical Collections, College of Physicians of Philadelphia.*

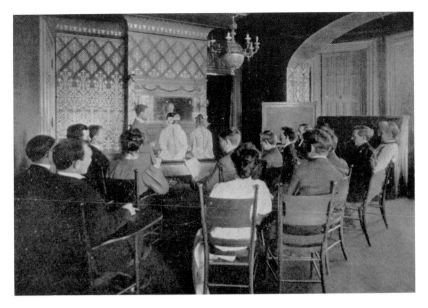

PRACTICAL ANATOMY GAVE students "hands-on" experience in the dissecting room. In the late eighteenth century the cadavers used by medical students were often supplied by grave-robbers or obtained through other irregular routes. Public distaste for such activity led to several attacks on the building at the Pennsylvania Hospital where dissections were performed. It also forced William Shippen, Jr. (1736–1808), an eighteenth-century lecturer in anatomy, to defend his work by explaining that he did not collect bodies from cemeteries but instead used the corpses of suicide victims, criminals, and, on occasion, indigents from the potter's field.

Despite vehement popular opposition, the practice of dissection grew in the mid-nineteenth century. In 1866 the law was changed to allow the dissection of unclaimed bodies. Gross or "practical" anatomy became a core subject in medical education. By the early twentieth century an ideal four-year medical course included 230 hours of laboratory anatomy during the first year and 60 hours the second year.

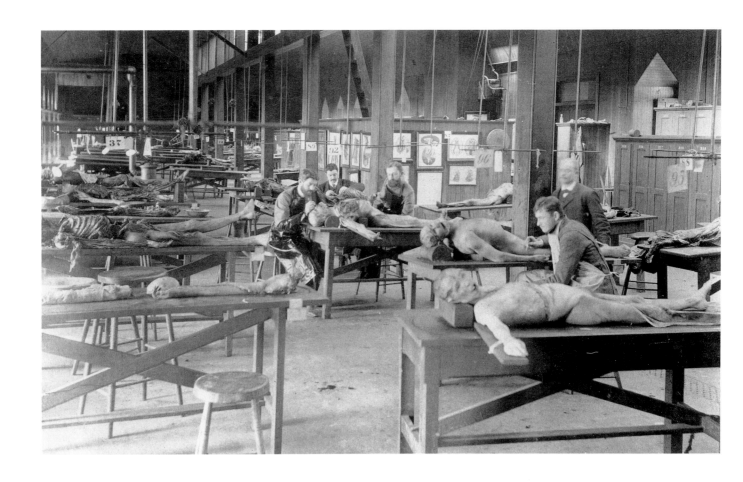

5.

Dissecting room, University of Pennsylvania School of Medicine. *University of Pennsylvania Archives.*

THE FIRST PHOTOGRAPH shows the dissecting room of the University of Pennsylvania School of Medicine in the mid-1880s.

The second is of the anatomy laboratory of the Temple University School of Medicine, which was then located over a stable. When the school opened in 1901 it offered a five-year evening course; in 1907 a four-year day program was adopted. The medical school was affiliated with the Samaritan Hospital, which, like Temple University, was founded by Baptist leader Russell H. Conwell (1843–1925).

10

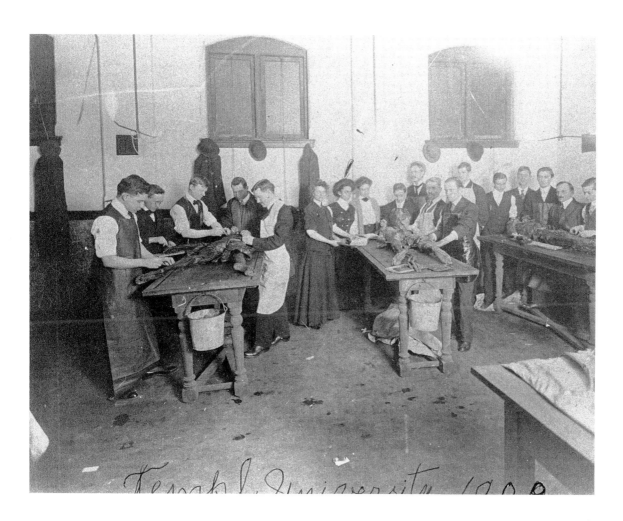

6.

Anatomy laboratory,
Temple University School
of Medicine.
*Conwellana-Templana
Collection, Temple
University.*

7.

Black medical students with cadaver, University of Pennsylvania School of Medicine.
I. Maximillian Martin.

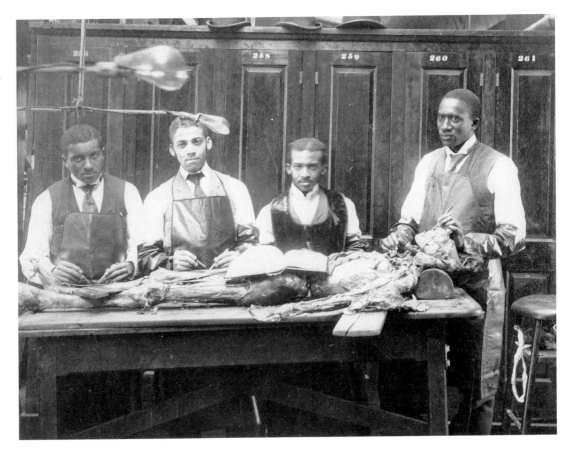

FOUR BLACK MEDICAL students are shown dissecting a cadaver in this 1896 photograph. Segregation and discrimination by race and gender were common features of medical education. Although black and female students were eventually admitted to all Philadelphia's medical schools, their number was carefully limited and they faced hostility throughout their careers.

Shown in this photograph are (left to right): Samuel Patterson Stafford, who practiced medicine in St. Louis for more than fifty years; Eugene Theodore Hinson (1873–1960), one of the founders of Philadelphia's Mercy Hospital, who served as chief of its gynecology service; Samuel Clifford Boston (1871–1924), who practiced medicine in Philadelphia; and Francis Julius Le Moyne Johnson (1870–1905), who practiced medicine in Washington, Pennsylvania.

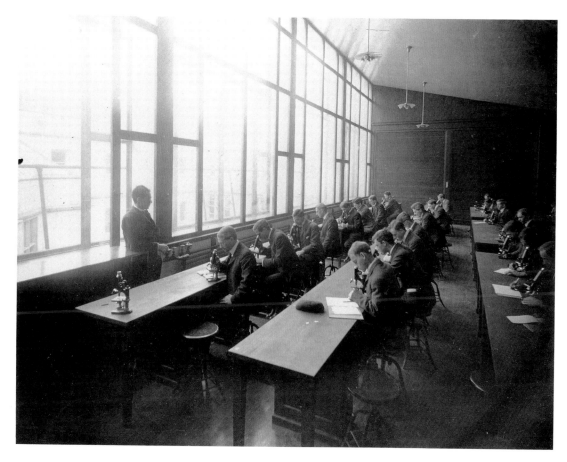

8.

Students at microscopes, surgical pathology laboratory, University of Pennsylvania School of Medicine.
University of Pennsylvania Archives.

THE INTRODUCTION OF laboratory teaching was a central aspect of reform in medical education. After the turn of the century, leading medical schools began increasing the number of science hours required for graduation. Following publication of the Carnegie-funded Flexner Report of 1910, which further emphasized reform of the medical school by setting ideal requirements for scientific and clinical training, chemistry, physiology, pharmacology, and bacteriology, became standard features of medical education.

Here students are at work in the surgical pathology laboratory of the University of Pennsylvania School of Medicine in the newly completed medical laboratory building in 1904. The state-of-the-art science building was designed with large windows to provide a light source for the microscopes and included, as one contemporary described it, "other more artificial accessories" to supply additional illumination.

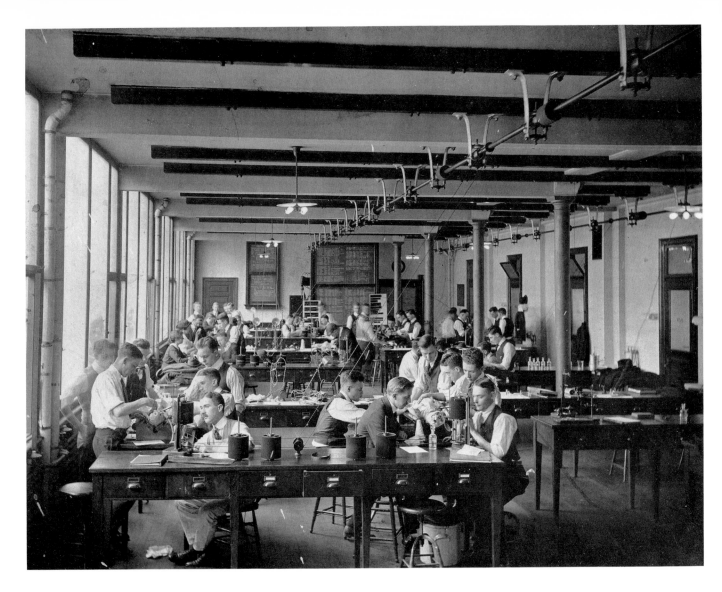

9.

Experimenting on animals in pharmacology laboratory, University of Pennsylvania School of Medicine.
University of Pennsylvania Archives.

OVER THE COURSE of the twentieth century laboratory science grew more sophisticated and was integrated more systematically into the curriculum. Pictured here is the pharmacology laboratory at the University of Pennsylvania School of Medicine in the 1920s. Students are conducting experiments (possibly measuring the effects of drugs on respiration or blood pressure) on animals. The results are being recorded on a kymograph.

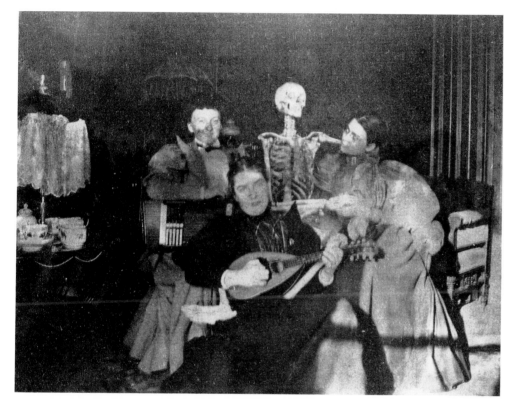

10.

Medical students with skeleton, Woman's Medical College.
Archives and Special Collections on Women in Medicine, The Medical College of Pennsylvania.

THERE WAS MORE to medical school life than lectures and study, as suggested in this photograph of three students (Nellie Louise Laurence, Ellen James Patterson, and Alice Hatheway Purvis-Robie) from the Woman's Medical College relaxing in their room in the mid-1890s. The photograph comes from the album of Laura Heath Hills, a student from 1892–1896 who practiced medicine in Connecticut for many decades.

Medical education for women in regular medical schools began in 1848 with the admission of Elizabeth Blackwell (1821–1910) to the Geneva Medical College; however, few regular institutions accepted "females" before the turn of the century, and those that did severely limited admissions. The majority of female practitioners were graduates of the five women's medical colleges founded by 1900.

Although the Woman's Medical College opened in 1850 (as the Female Medical College of Pennsylvania), its graduates were not recognized by the state medical society until 1871, despite the fact that the education they received was comparable to or better than that given to the graduates of Pennsylvania's male institutions. In 1969, after graduating over 3,000 women physicians, the school became coeducational.

11.

Physiology laboratory,
University of Pennsyl-
vania School of Medicine.
*University of Pennsyl-
vania Archives.*

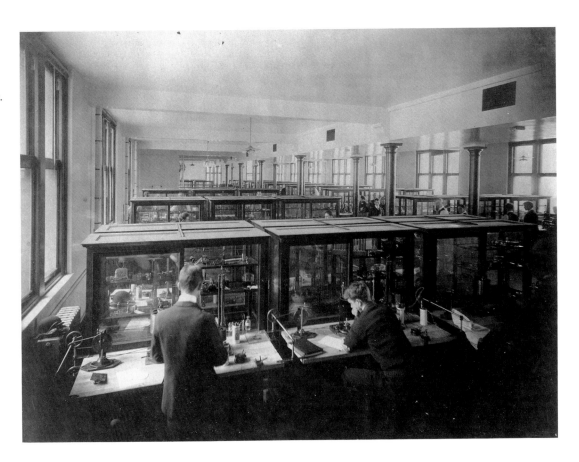

BY THE FIRST decade of the twentieth century, preclinical laboratory study and bedside training were accepted by America's "better schools," as key elements in medical education. The professors who chaired the preclinical departments no longer had to earn their living in clinical practice, but instead received salaries that allowed them to engage in full-time teaching and some research. With more curriculum time devoted to laboratory study and research, additional facilities were necessary, and in 1904 a new medical laboratory building opened at the University of Pennsylvania. It provided what historian George Corner called "roomy modern quarters including ample space for research" in laboratories dedicated to physiology, pathology, and pharmacology.

The first image shows the physiology laboratory in 1904; the second and third, also from 1904, come from the pharmacology laboratory and the museum of the pathology department; the fourth is the bacteriology laboratory, photographed in 1908.

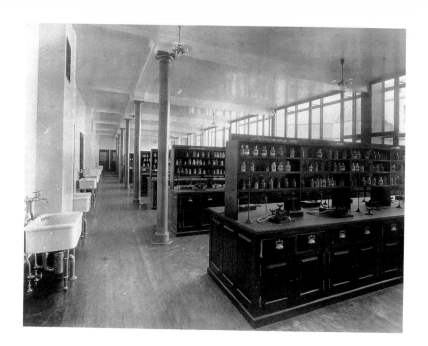

12.

Pharmacology laboratory, University of Pennsylvania School of Medicine. *University of Pennsylvania Archives.*

13.

Museum of Pathology, University of Pennsylvania School of Medicine. *University of Pennsylvania Archives.*

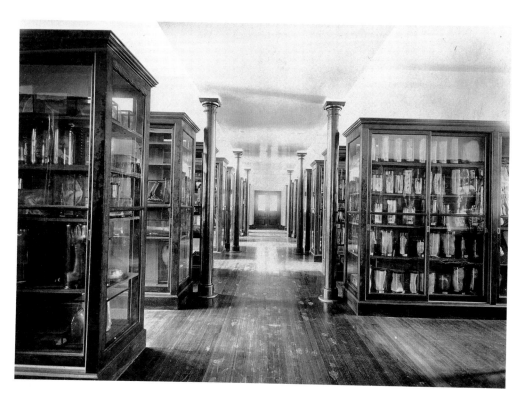

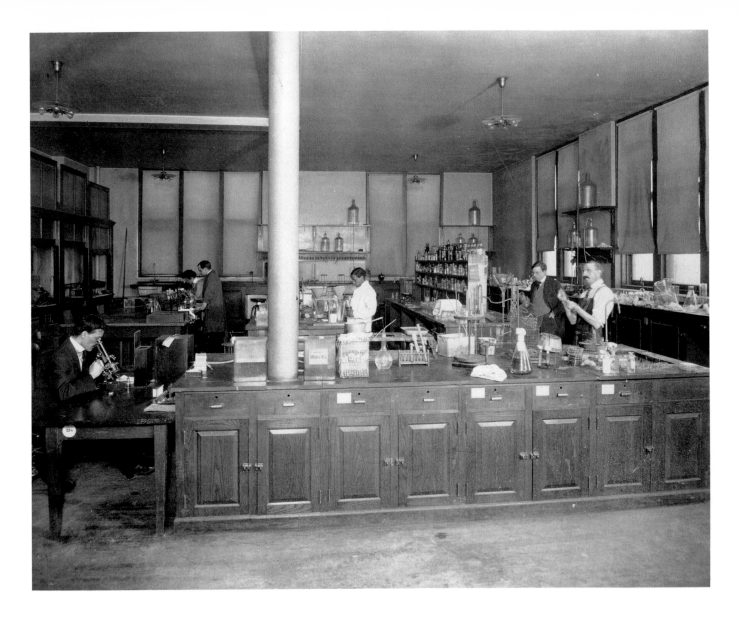

14.

Bacteriology laboratory,
University of Pennsyl-
vania School of Medicine.
*University of Pennsyl-
vania Archives.*

Perhaps the most dramatic moment of initiation into clinical training came when the student had an opportunity to observe his or her first surgical operation. This same excitement attracted successive generations of photographers to the hospital's surgical amphitheater. The images they recorded illustrate the increasingly sterile conditions in which operations were performed and the growing technical complexity of the procedures undertaken.

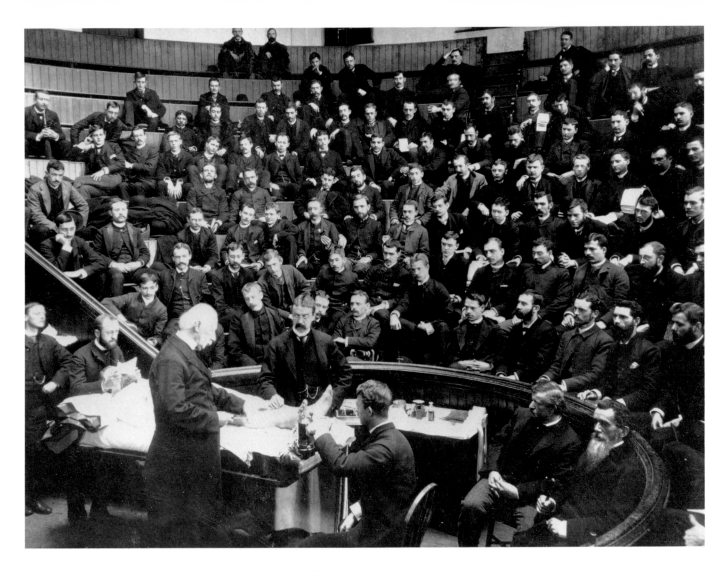

15.

Agnew performing a leg
operation, University of
Pennsylvania School of
Medicine.
University of Pennsylvania Archives.

IN THIS PHOTOGRAPH from 1886, possibly the
model for the famous painting by Thomas Eakins,
Dr. D. Hayes Agnew (1818–1892) of the University of Pennsylvania School of Medicine performs
a leg operation under the watchful eyes of numerous medical students. Agnew and his assistants
are dressed in street clothes. Anesthesia is being
administered through an ether cone.

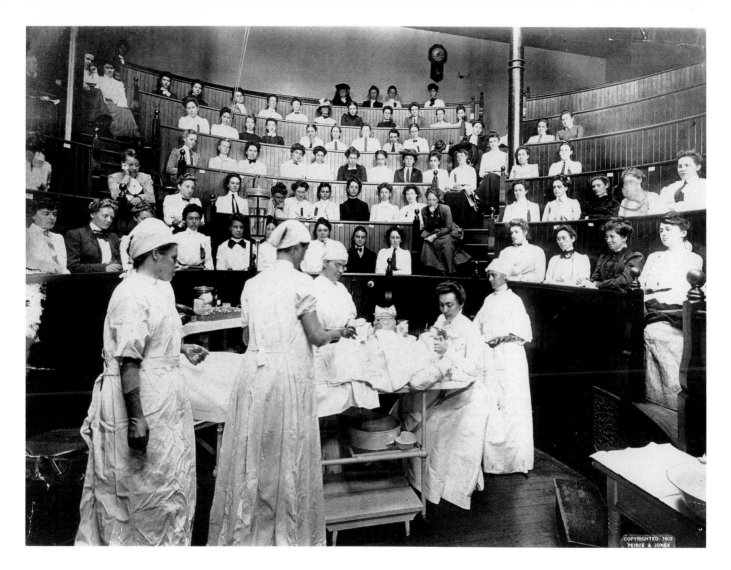

EARLY ASEPTIC CONDITIONS prevail in this 1903 operation at the Woman's Medical College of Pennsylvania. The physicians are gloved and gowned and, with the exception of the anesthesiologist, they are wearing caps. Instruments would have been sterilized in an autoclave. At this time anesthesia was not yet a recognized specialty; junior residents or attending physicians might serve as anesthesiologist, and it was assumed that all house officers should become familiar with this useful skill. Aseptic procedures (which sought to keep bacteria from coming into contact with wounds or incisions) had evolved dramatically from their origins in Joseph Lister's (1827–1912) experimental "antiseptic" procedures of the 1860s.

16.

Surgeons in operating room, Woman's Medical College.
Archives and Special Collections on Women in Medicine, The Medical College of Pennsylvania.

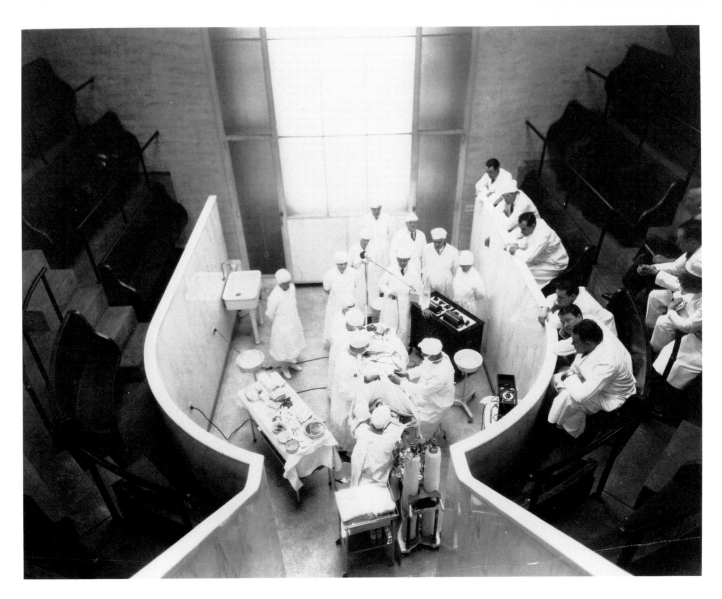

17.

Surgery in amphitheater,
Philadelphia General
Hospital.
*Center for the Study of
the History of Nursing,
School of Nursing, Uni-
versity of Pennsylvania.*

TAKEN IN THE Philadelphia General Hospital surgical amphitheater, this 1929 photograph shows
the surgeons wearing masks. Those without
masks were members of the radiology department, suggesting that this might have been a
cancer operation.

IF THE STUDENT'S first visit to the surgical amphitheater provided the most dramatic introduction to the hospital, observations in the clinics and on the wards provided his or her practical introduction to medical work. Peering over someone's shoulder or standing beside the physician, students observed not only the techniques of physical diagnosis but what we have come to call interpersonal skills. It is difficult to know whether the patients, surrounded by students and interns, found the experience actively intrusive, a routine to be assumed and expected, or perhaps even a novel interruption of the ward's dreary routine. Clinic and ward patients were, after all, expected to serve as "teaching material."

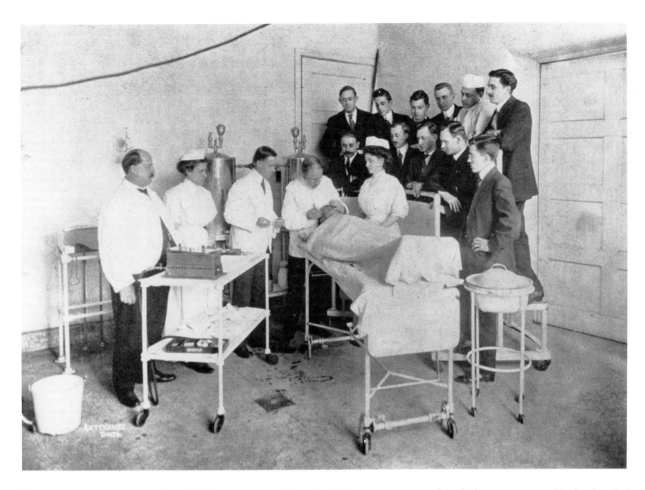

18.

Students observing in eye
sub-clinic, Hahnemann
Hospital.
*Archives, Hahnemann
University.*

THIS 1910 PHOTOGRAPH from the Hahnemann
Hospital eye sub-clinic shows eleven students observing a physician at work. Lying on a stretcher,
the patient appears to be undergoing a surgical
procedure, rather than just a simple examination.
Ophthalmology was one of the earliest medical
specialties. Inpatient ophthalmology beds and
outpatient services proliferated in late-nineteenth-
century general hospitals, while ophthalmology

hospitals were among England and America's earliest specialty institutions.

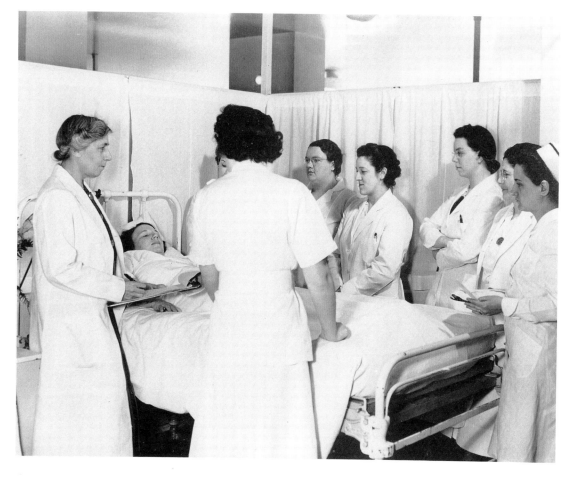

19.

Clinical rounds at Woman's Medical College. *Archives and Special Collections on Women in Medicine, The Medical College of Pennsylvania.*

IN THIS SCENE, familiar to any late-twentieth-century patient in a teaching hospital, students stand around the patient's bed listening to the attending physician discuss the case. Clinical rounds—in which attending physicians, residents, and medical students move from bed to bed in the wards or rooms discussing the diagnosis and management of each case—is one of the fundamental elements in medical education. An ideal goal of would-be educational reformers at mid-nineteenth century, it had become routine by the First World War.

The students in this photograph, taken in 1942 at the Hospital of the Woman's Medical College, have assumed the same serious and respectful demeanor as those depicted in the previous photograph—despite all the medical, technological, and bureaucratic changes in the intervening years.

20.

Physicians examining
x-ray images, University
of Pennsylvania School of
Medicine.
*University of Pennsyl-
vania Archives.*

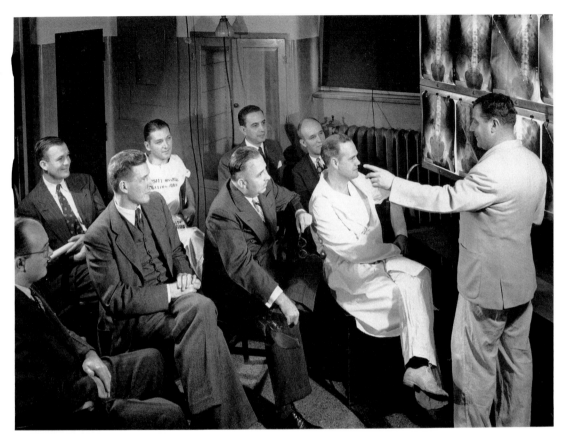

PROGRESS IN SCIENTIFIC medicine made new kinds
of information available. Increasingly, physicians
relied upon laboratory tests, electrocardiograms,
and x-rays to reveal mechanisms underlying a
patient's presenting complaint. When first intro-
duced, these new technologies were used infre-
quently, sometimes out of mere curiosity rather
than as a means of providing day-to-day clinical
guidance. But as the value of these diagnostic
procedures became known, they were applied
with greater frequency. The review of such tests

became an important part of the house officer's
education.

Surgeons obtained invaluable information from
x-rays. In this image, Professor of Surgery I. S.
Ravdin (1894–1972) is reviewing x-rays. Ravdin,
a distinguished teacher, was Harrison Professor of
Surgery and, later, the University of Pennsylvania's Vice-President for Medical Affairs.

For DOCTORS IN training, the introduction to a community came through a local dispensary. In this photograph from 1916 a physician from the Woman's Medical College Hospital is visiting patients living off an alleyway only a block from the hospital dispensary, located in north Philadelphia.

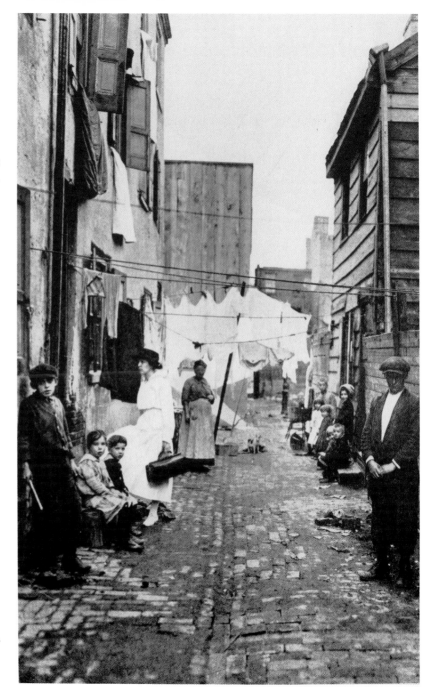

21.

Physician from Woman's Medical College Hospital visiting patients. *Archives and Special Collections on Women in Medicine, The Medical College of Pennsylvania.*

22.

Residents' room, Pennsylvania Hospital.
Archives of Pennsylvania Hospital.

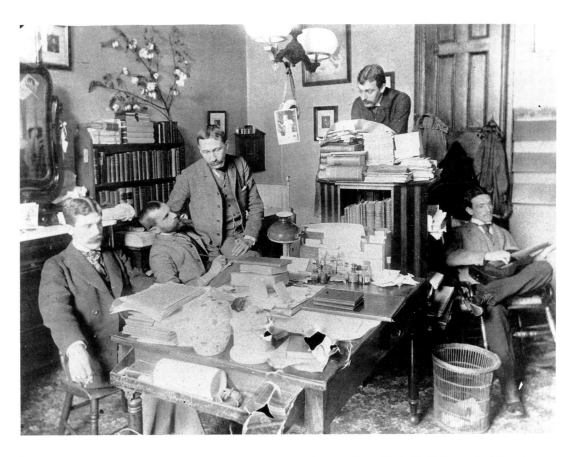

IN THE LATE NINETEENTH century, patronage was the key to obtaining a position as a hospital house officer. But once having secured one of these posts, young physicians found themselves working long hours with no remuneration beyond board and room; they were repaid in the form of clinical experience and professional credentials.

The house officers pictured here in the residents' room at the Pennsylvania Hospital seem to be "gentlemen" in appearance—and in all likelihood in reality as well. They were indeed selected in part because of their social status and the patronage it implied. Until the end of the nineteenth century, the Pennsylvania Hospital's lay Board of Managers, recruited from among the city's prominent families, exercised ultimate authority in the selection of house officers.

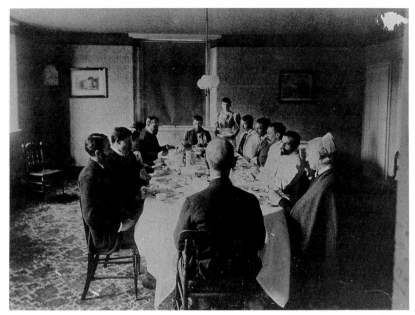

23.

Dining room, Pennsyl-
vania Hospital.
*Archives of Pennsylvania
Hospital.*

24.

Administrative staff and
others, Philadelphia Gen-
eral Hospital.
*Center for the Study of
the History of Nursing,
School of Nursing, Uni-
versity of Pennsylvania.*

WITHIN THE EARLY hospital, day-to-day management was delegated to a lay superintendent who
bore a paternal responsibility for the institution
and its inmates. The superintendent ordinarily
lived in the hospital with his own family, and his
wife served as matron, in charge of servants,
food, and laundry. The apothecary and the house
staff ate at the superintendent's table. An undated
image (possibly from the 1880s) taken in the basement dining room of the Pennsylvania Hospital
provides a compelling view of the hospital staff as
extended family.

A more formal portrait from the Philadelphia
General Hospital in 1885 includes the steward,
standing on the far left, the druggist, standing on
the far right, Alice Fisher (1839–1888), the first
superintendent of the hospital's nursing school,
seated in the front row, as well as several of the
residents and nurses.

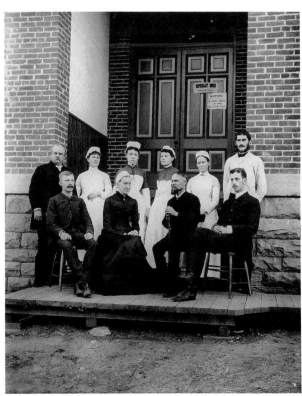

25.

Stricken physician in bed, Philadelphia General Hospital.
Historical Collections, College of Physicians of Philadelphia.

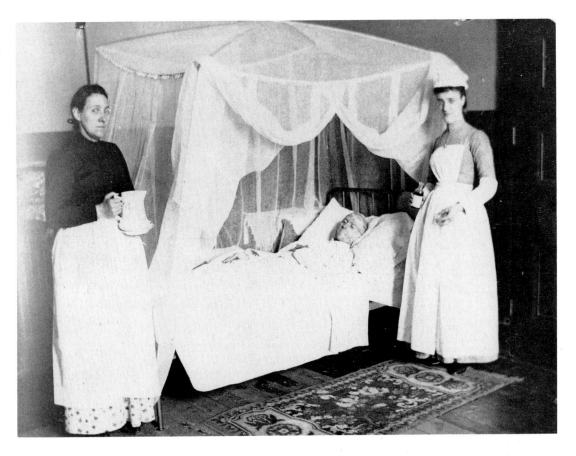

EMBARKING ON A resident house officership marked the passage from student to practitioner and was accompanied by new risks. Physicians contracted infectious diseases from their patients, and some of these ills proved disabling or deadly. Tuberculosis, for example, was a frequent assailant of both student physicians and nurses.

For those who were stricken, hospitals maintained special beds and wards. The first image shows Dr. James Wardlaw Pelham (1861?–1906), an 1888 resident of the Philadelphia General

Hospital. The second, from the Hospital of the University of Pennsylvania in 1907, records the well-maintained student ward. Despite its fine furnishings, it is a hospital ward nonetheless, and for those being treated it constituted the site of an all too personal encounter with disease.

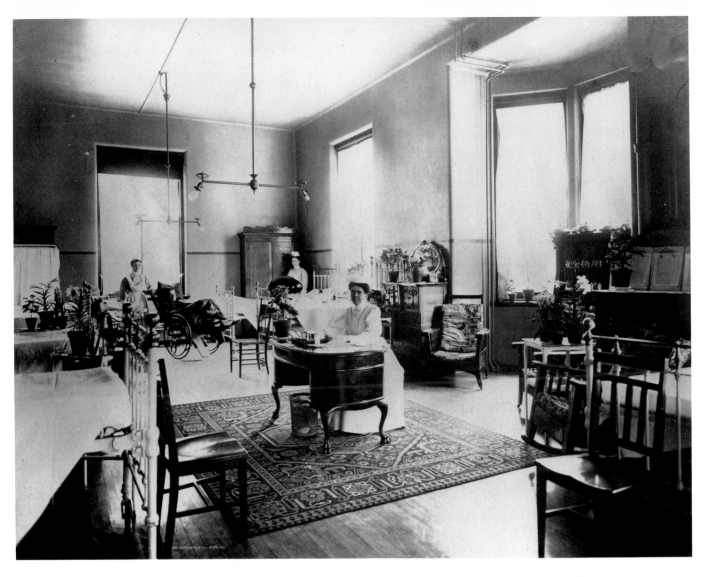

26.

Student ward, Hospital
of the University of
Pennsylvania.
*University of Pennsyl-
vania Archives.*

27.

Interns, Woman's Hospital of Philadelphia. *Archives and Special Collections on Women in Medicine, The Medical College of Pennsylvania.*

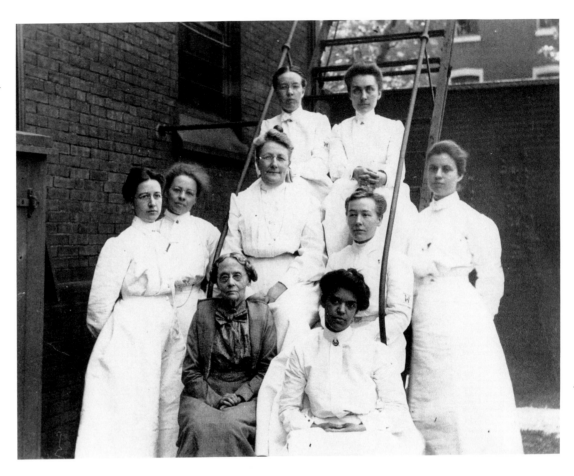

IN THE HOSPITAL, the isolation of medical school life, defined by the need to study written texts, gave way to the demands of living texts, the ward's patients, and taskmasters in the person of supervising physicians. Despite long hours on duty, those employed in the hospital seem to have had, as these photographs show, enormous pride in their work and in earning the designation "doctor."

In the first image, the interns of the Woman's Hospital of Philadelphia for the year 1903–1904

pose outside the hospital in their uniforms. Opened in 1861, the Woman's Hospital of Philadelphia was the city's oldest hospital serving women and children. Equally important, it offered facilities for clinical instruction to women physicians and also maintained a nurse training school. Among those in the photograph are Ellen C. Potter (1871–1958) (top left), who served as Commissioner of Health for the Commonwealth of Pennsylvania, and Lillie Rosa Minoka-Hill (1876–1952) (bottom

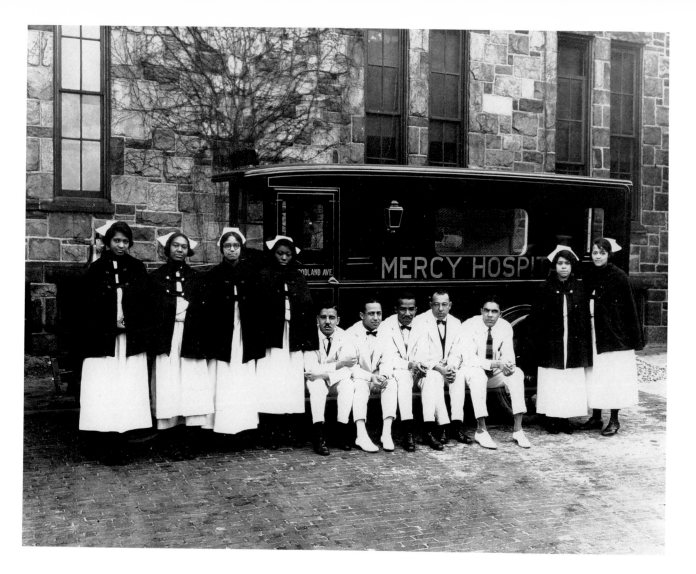

right), who practiced medicine in Oneida,
Wisconsin.

In the second image, the residents and nurses
of the Mercy Hospital and School for Nurses
circa 1930 pose beside the ambulance—a favorite
backdrop for such pictures. The Mercy Hospital
and School for Nurses, Philadelphia's second
black hospital, opened in 1907.

28.

Residents and nurses,
Mercy Hospital.
*Center for the Study of
the History of Nursing,
School of Nursing, Uni-
versity of Pennsylvania.*

THE TRAINED NURSE, a graduate of one of the many hospital nursing schools that developed in the last two decades of the nineteenth century, commenced her education by caring for patients under the direction of a nursing supervisor and a cadre of experienced ward nurses. It was hard work. The Hahnemann Hospital rule book for the 1890s, typical for its era, noted that day nurses were on duty from 7 A.M. to 8 P.M. with a half hour off duty for dinner. Night nurses were on duty from 8 P.M. to 7 A.M. The nurses performed both housekeeping and nursing tasks but were strictly forbidden from doing the doctors' sewing or mending. For their labor they received room, board, laundry (limited to eighteen pieces each week including bed linen), and a small stipend to cover the costs of books and clothing. Hahnemann and other hospitals gained much in return from their staff of trained and student nurses. Without them, hospitals would never have become acceptable to middle-class patients, nor could they have maintained the kind of discipline and order necessary to the provision of an increasingly technical medical care.

Hospital schools provided classroom instruction as well, and the didactic and scientific portion of nursing education was to increase dramatically during the twentieth century. Nevertheless, it was the knowledge gained on the job that gave the trained nurse her credentials in the eyes of patients who hired graduates to care for them at home. When the market for trained nurses—especially for private duty—began to diminish in the twenties and thirties, nursing leaders sought ways to upgrade the profession. They argued for limitations on the production of nurses and the need to emphasize classroom training in science, rather than in skills gained at the bedside. Opposing this view were some physicians and others who believed that practice, not theory, should dominate the nursing curriculum.

Until the mid-1930s most trained nurses found careers in private-duty nursing; only a small elite found situations as nursing school superintendents, and a larger minority occupied full-time hospital staff positions. But after the Great Depression left thousands of nurses without work, many sought hospital employment. During the same years, many hospitals closed their nurse training schools as they discovered it was cheaper to hire graduate nurses than maintain student nurses. Hospitals became the chief employer of trained nurses.

The composition of the trained nurse labor force changed over time, reflecting both the options available to women seeking careers and the pay and status accorded the nursing profession. Initially nurse training schools attracted many young, native-born, single women, often from rural areas; a not insignificant minority at the better schools came from middle-class backgrounds and boasted solid academic credentials. Later nursing students were drawn from a wider pool that included the daughters of immigrants, blacks, and the urban working class. What remained consistent was the ideology of caring, the belief that nurses performed a rewarding service to others. This belief shaped expectations of nurses and those who employed them, at times serving to discourage nurses from articulating demands for economic and professional acknowledgment.

While photographers flocked to hospital amphitheaters to record the charismatic surgeons wielding their attention-focusing knives, the nurses they found there and elsewhere were peripheral to the dramatic structure of these cliched images. The dichotomies of gender—male physicians, female nurses—and of health services—caring and curing—ensured that the young women found in most such photographs were marginal to the conventionally staged tableau, if not to the actual activity it was presumed to record. Still we do have a few images that show nurses without patients: in the classroom, in the dormitory, at graduation, and posed decorously in manicured ward settings.

29.

Nurses collecting soiled
dressings, Pennsylvania
Hospital.
*Archives of Pennsylvania
Hospital.*

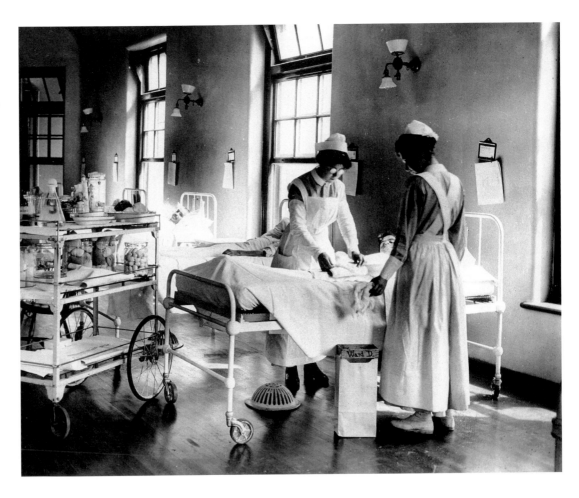

THE GROWTH OF nurse training schools in the
United States reflected and facilitated the expansion of general hospitals. The first three nurse
training schools opened in 1872 and 1873; twenty
years later there were over 400, and by 1920 there
were 1,700. Despite the long hours, the seven-
day work week, and the strict discipline, many
women sought training and the opportunity to ac-
quire a skill.

According to one estimate, between 98 and 99
percent of nursing education in the 1890s consisted of practical work. A photograph of nurses
at work in the 1890s is necessarily a photograph
of nursing education as well. In the first image,
circa 1900, nurses at the Pennsylvania Hospital
move through Ward D, collecting soiled dressings. In the second image from the same era, two
students at the Philadelphia General Hospital

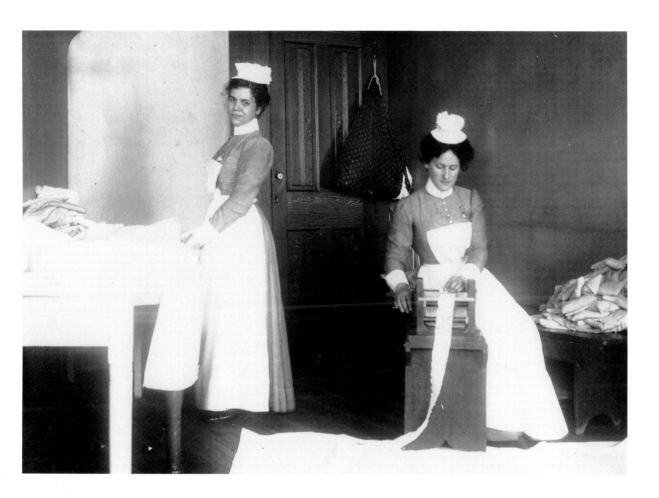

School of Nursing—Susannah Fisher (class of 1891) and Florence Ingram (class of 1889)—demonstrate the rolling of bandages.

By the 1920s, educational standards had been raised and the Standard Curriculum for Schools of Nursing, prepared by the National League of Nursing Education, was revised and expanded to reflect the on-going effort by nursing leaders to improve the quality of both clinical and theo-retical training. Among the subjects studied by nursing school students were anatomy, physi-ology, chemistry, bacteriology, therapeutics, hygiene, and dietetics. The time devoted to each subject varied a good deal; the least ambitious schools demanded, in fact, very little in the way of classroom work from their students.

30.

Nurses rolling bandages in workroom, Phila-delphia General Hospital. *Center for the Study of the History of Nursing, School of Nursing, University of Pennsylvania.*

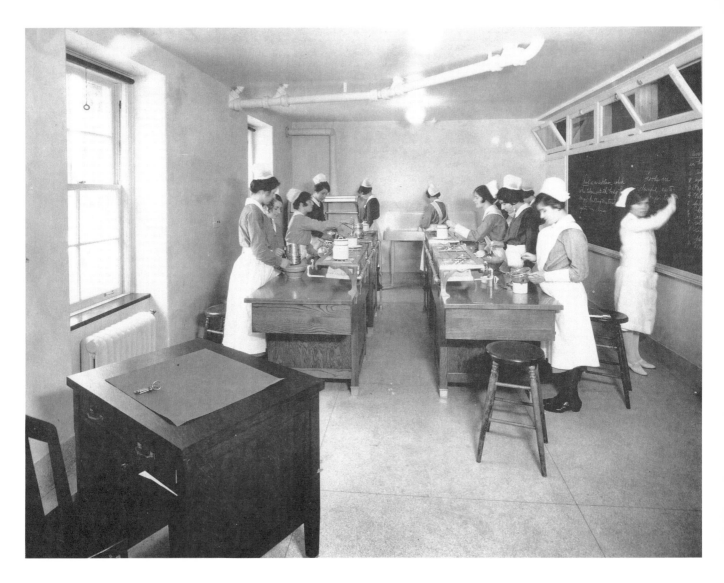

31.

Chestnut Hill Hospital nurses in nutrition class. *Center for the Study of the History of Nursing, School of Nursing, University of Pennsylvania.*

IN THIS 1927 picture from the Chestnut Hill Hospital, students are shown in the classroom studying nutrition. The subject encompassed the general effects of food on health and in recuperation, as well as the preparation of specific diets considered important in certain illnesses such as typhoid.

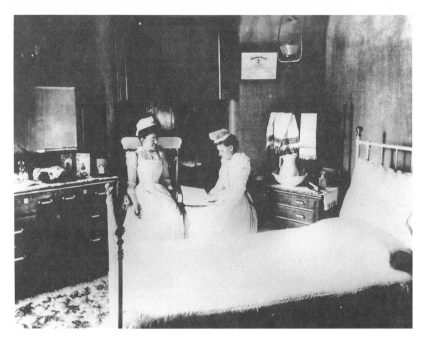

When America's first nurse training schools opened in the last quarter of the nineteenth century, students lived in the hospital, but eventually separate residences became standard. While nursing school brochures and annual reports were sometimes illustrated with photographs showing pleasant, well-furnished surroundings, the recollections of the nurses make it clear that accommodations were far from luxurious and often overcrowded. The following images seem posed and were in all likelihood intended to "advertise" their respective nursing schools to potential applicants.

In the first, taken in 1887, two nurses from Pennsylvania Hospital are shown in their room. In the second, taken at the Philadelphia General Hospital circa 1910, three off-duty nurses enjoy some relaxing moments in the parlor. The Nurses' Home at Philadelphia General Hospital was erected in 1895. Prior to that time nurses lived in cramped quarters within the hospital, described by Superintendent Charles Lawrence in 1900 as "little cubbies erected in the wards."

32.

Nurses in their room, Pennsylvania Hospital. *Archives of Pennsylvania Hospital.*

33.

Nurses in parlor, Philadelphia General Hospital. *Center for the Study of the History of Nursing, School of Nursing, University of Pennsylvania.*

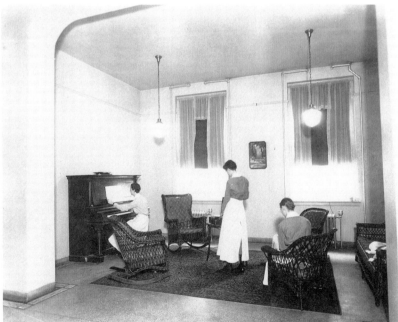

34.

Nurses playing in wheel-
barrow, Philadelphia
General Hospital.
*Center for the Study of
the History of Nursing,
School of Nursing, Uni-
versity of Pennsylvania.*

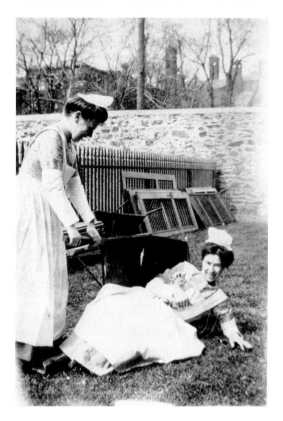

DESPITE THE LONG hours on the ward there was
still time to play, as these more informal photographs indicate. In the first, taken at the Philadelphia General Hospital soon after the turn of the
century, two nurses in uniform are enjoying some
respite from their duties. The picture comes from
the album of Robert J. Hunter (1882–1980) a hospital resident from 1904 to 1906.

The other photograph shows nurses from St.
Luke's Homeopathic Hospital and Dispensary
standing outside the institution in 1911. It was
taken by Marie Louise Bormann (1887–1918),
who trained at St. Luke's as well as at St. Timo-
thy's Memorial Hospital and House of Mercy in
Roxborough.

In some ways these pictures of the nurses off
duty are as misleading as the ones showing them
posed stiffly in the parlor; for most nurses work
was the dominant activity. At St. Luke's, for example, between four and six students entered the
three-year program each year and provided the
bulk of the care for a sixty-bed hospital.

35.

Group of nurses outside
St. Luke's Hospital.
*Historical Society of
Pennsylvania.*

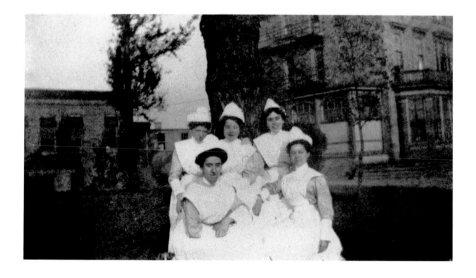

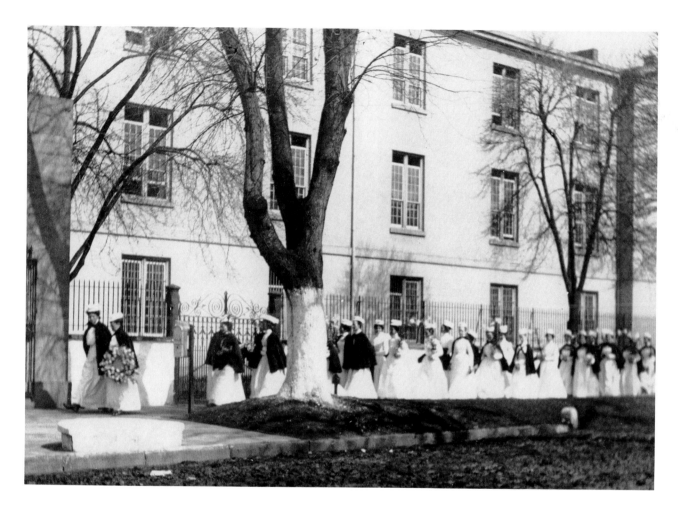

GRADUATES OF HOSPITAL nursing schools wore the uniforms and caps and pins of their training institution on their private-duty assignments or while serving as superintendents of other institutions. The awarding of that cap constituted an important ritual.

Nursing schools had other rituals as well. At the Philadelphia General Hospital it was an Easter Sunday tradition for the student nurses and alumnae to walk in uniform to the nearby Woodlands Cemetery to visit the grave of Alice Fisher, the first Chief Nurse and director of the training school. Here is the annual "white parade" in 1900, headed by Marion E. Smith (d. 1943), Chief Nurse, and Lydia A. Whiton, her assistant.

36.

Nurses on parade, Philadelphia General Hospital. *Center for the Study of the History of Nursing, School of Nursing, University of Pennsylvania.*

37.

Graduates, Mercy Hospital School for Nurses. *Historical Society of Pennsylvania.*

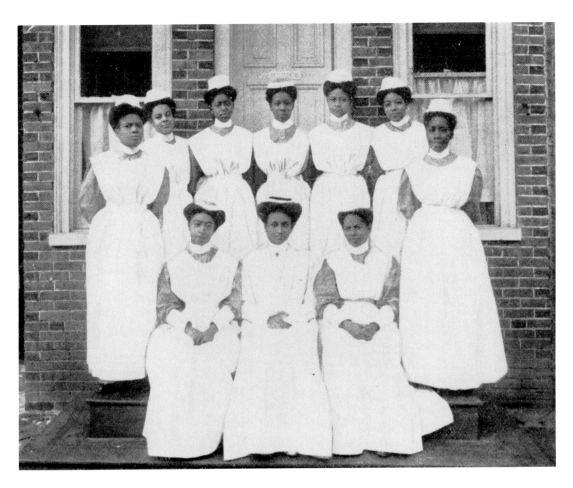

GRADUATION NOT ONLY marked the completion of training, but conferred upon women the status of trained professionals, ready to serve the public. The pride of the graduates can be seen in this image from the Mercy Hospital School for Nurses. Between 1907 and 1950 the school graduated 386 trained nurses. Along with Philadelphia's Frederick Douglass Hospital, Mercy Hospital offered one of the few hospital training schools available to black women who sought professional training.

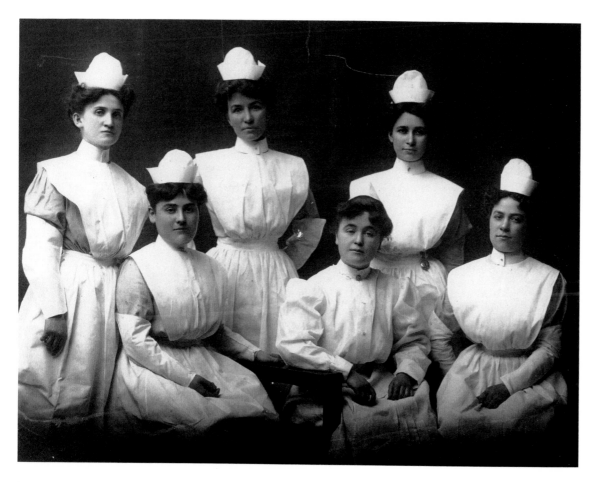

THE SAME SENSE of self-respect and pride can be seen in the first graduating class from Mt. Sinai Hospital (known today as Einstein Southern Division) in 1908. The hospital, located in the densely populated southeastern section of the city, was originally organized by the Beth Israel Hospital Association to offer medical and surgical services to Philadelphia's sick Jewish poor.

38.

Mt. Sinai Hospital nursing school graduates. *Balch Institute Library.*

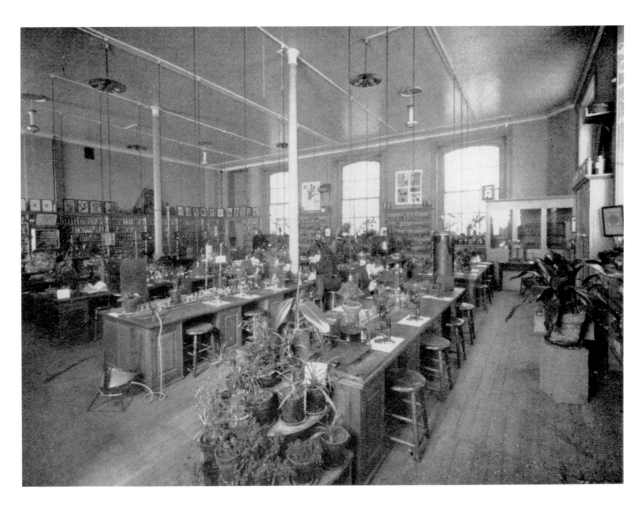

39.

Students in laboratory, Philadelphia College of Pharmacy.
Historical Collection, College of Physicians of Philadelphia.

IN ADDITION TO the physicians and nurses shown above, large numbers of other health professionals obtained their training in Philadelphia. Some received their education within separate institutions, such as schools of dentistry, pharmacy, podiatry, and optometry.

The Philadelphia College of Pharmacy, America's first such institution, incorporated in 1822, remains in operation to this day. It provided for-

mal (as opposed to apprenticeship) training in the compounding and dispensing of drugs. Some of its graduates managed hospital pharmacies; a far greater proportion worked in their own shops, where they filled a variety of health care needs. This photograph shows one of the school's laboratories in 1910. The plants were almost certainly used to demonstrate the source of pharmaceuticals.

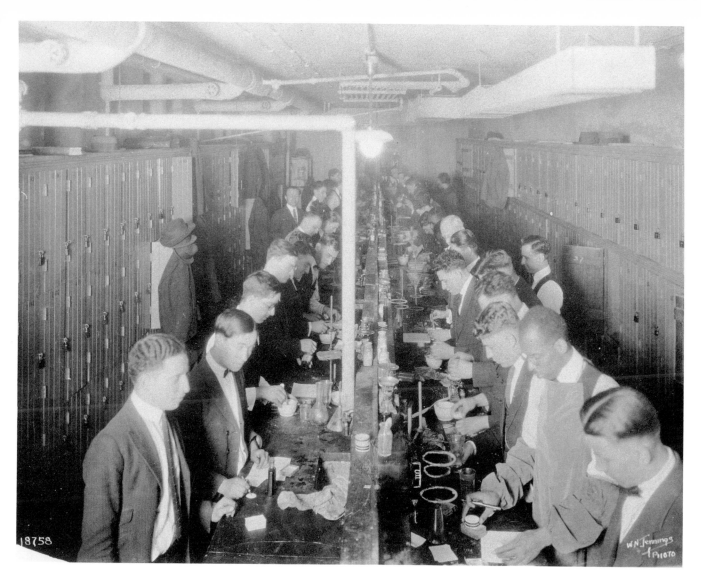

WHILE THE COLLEGE of Pharmacy began in opposition to the plan of the University of Pennsylvania to create a pharmacy program, the Temple University's School of Pharmacy began within the School of Medicine. In 1905 it became an independent school within the university. Shown here are students in the school's laboratory in 1912.

40.

Pharmacy students, Temple University. *Conwellana-Templana Collection, Temple University.*

TWO

Hospitals:
The Delivery of
Medical Care

THE PROLIFERATION OF hospitals in late-nineteenth- and early-twentieth-century Philadelphia reflected urban demography as much as it did a need for care and the desire to provide for clinical education. Both the pride and interest of the city's varied racial, ethnic, and religious communities were manifested in the construction of hospitals—while the ever-increasing scale of Philadelphia General Hospital mirrored the growing burden of dependency that paralleled the city's growth in wealth and in population.

Despite their varied sponsorship, the hospital had, by the 1920s, become an important part of the medical care system, for the middle class as well as the poor and dependent who had constituted its exclusive clientele a half-century earlier. And much of that inpatient care was delivered on a fee-for-service basis; in 1875 no Philadelphia attending physician routinely submitted a bill for hospital care he (or in a few instances she) had provided. Philadelphians able to pay a physician's fees would not willingly have sought treatment in a hospital bed.

Photographs were taken in the hospital for many reasons. Some were efforts to document the "good works" of the hospital's wards and clinics; others advertised the comfort of private rooms and the reassuringly white and gleaming operating and delivery rooms. Middle-class Americans had to be convinced that the hospital offered technical resources that could not be matched in a private home. Some images appeared in annual reports and other official documents; a few, such as some of those reproduced in the special section on the Philadelphia General Hospital, were taken by hospital interns recording the milieu in which they studied, worked, and relaxed. In many cases the photographer and the intended purpose of the photograph are unknown, but collectively the images convey the emergence of a modern medical institution.

41.

Frederick Douglass Memorial Hospital and Training School for Nurses.
Afro-American Historical and Cultural Museum.

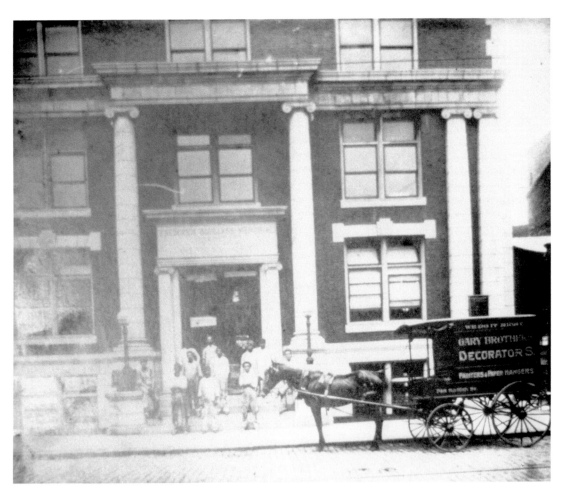

IN 1895 DR. Nathan Francis Mossell, the first black graduate of the University of Pennsylvania Medical School, opened the Frederick Douglass Memorial Hospital and Training School for Nurses. Located on Lombard and Sixteenth Streets in the heart of the city's black neighborhood, the hospital as shown here occupied a small building. In addition to offering care to neighborhood residents, Douglass was a professional training site, providing the only residency opportunities available to the city's black physicians as well as a training school for nurses. A second black hospital, the Mercy Hospital and Training School for Nurses, opened in Philadelphia in 1907. The opening of these two facilities reflected a national movement that saw the founding of approximately one hundred black hospitals in the period from 1890 to 1910.

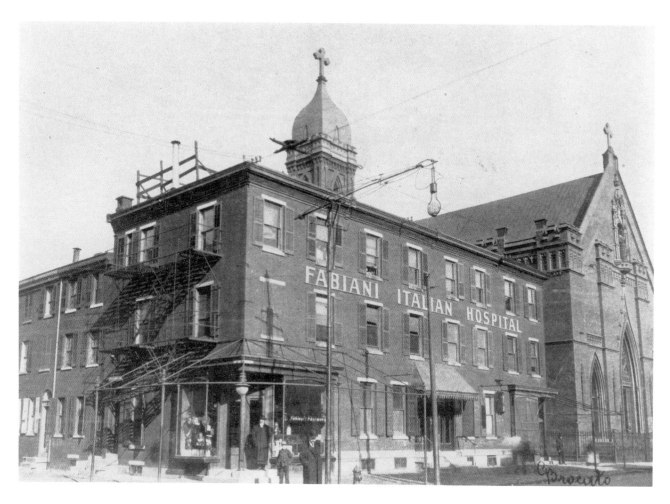

ETHNICITY, RELIGION, COMMUNITY need, sectarian diversity (most significantly homeopathy and osteopathy), and a trend toward specialization also led to the construction of new hospitals. The Fabiani Italian Hospital, founded in 1904 by Dr. Guiseppe Fabiani, stood at 10th and Christian Streets in South Philadelphia and served the immigrant Italian community that had established itself in the vicinity. Fabiani, an 1889 graduate of the University of Naples, emigrated to the United States in 1902.

42.

Fabiani Italian Hospital. *Balch Institute Library.*

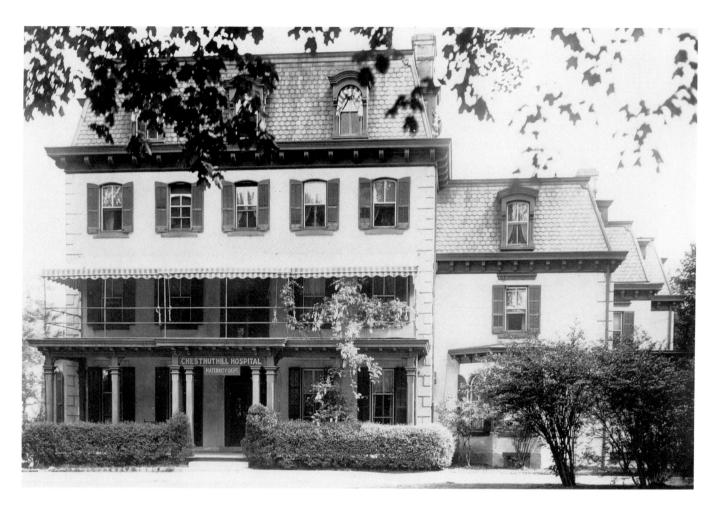

43.

Chestnut Hill Hospital.
*Center for the Study of
the History of Nursing,
School of Nursing, Uni-
versity of Pennsylvania.*

THE CHESTNUT HILL HOSPITAL, shown here in
1913, was located in the former private residence,
Norriton, of the Norris family of Chestnut Hill.
Lacking a hospital to serve emergency cases,
Chestnut Hill residents had to travel four miles to
the nearest facility before the hospital opened in
1904. Conversions of homes (often willed or donated for community purposes) into hospitals was

a frequent tactic in small towns and cities. The
photograph illustrates the relatively undifferenti-
ated quality of the hospital as physical artifact in
this period.

THE TRANSFORMATION OF hospitals from welfare
institutions serving the dependent into professional medical facilities was largely complete by
1920. Physical expansion and spatial differentiation were both necessary, as the hospital had
come to house not just the sick poor but laboratories, operating rooms, private suites, and wards
of various sorts. Along with these came the
mechanized laundries, institutional kitchens, and
other components of any modern institution.
Typical of the older hospital is Hahnemann,
shown here in 1925. In 1928 a new twenty-story,
735-bed hospital was erected and this building became the Medical College.

The history of Hahnemann Hospital is intertwined with that of Hahnemann Medical College.
At times they operated as separate institutions,
merging finally in 1885. The architecture of the
Hahnemann Hospital building shown here in 1925
is evocative of a church or temple and suggests
that the hospital functioned as an embodiment of
and monument to the new faith in scientific
medicine.

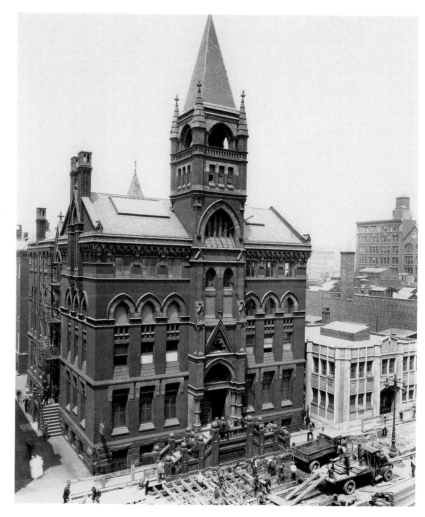

44.

Hahnemann University
Hospital.
*City Archives of
Philadelphia.*

BETWEEN 1880 AND 1920 the hospital had transformed itself. It not only was more specialized and more integrated into medical education, but also provided a different sort of care for a greater variety of Americans. And, whether delivered on a fee-for-service basis or received as charity, hospital care was almost certain to constitute a very different experience. Average stays grew shorter as surgery became increasingly significant and acute care came to dominate the hospital's image—and often its admissions. Trained nurses provided a new and bureaucratically structured style of care, both reassuring and distancing. And, of course, the technology almost absent from the nineteenth-century hospital had already come to symbolize and legitimate the twentieth-century hospital. Aseptic surgery, the x-ray, and clinical pathology laboratories had all become indispensable parts of the new model institution. A national system of accreditation, first developed in the era of World War I, acknowledged and enforced this reality.

DISPENSARIES AND CLINICS

MOST MEDICAL COMPLAINTS were treated by private practitioners, by physicians in free-standing community dispensaries, or in the later decades of the twentieth century in hospital clinics and emergency rooms. Facilities for inpatient care, although often photographed, accounted for only a portion of the institutional care provided in Philadelphia.

Dispensaries and clinics met the needs of physicians as well as patients, providing medical students the opportunity to learn by observation and recent graduates a chance to practice and improve their skills. In the nineteenth century, before required internships or formal specialized residencies, such outpatient posts provided the functional equivalents of advanced training programs for bright young physicians. The working-class patients who patronized these outpatient units rarely had the resources to pay for private care—and almost never for the specialist's costly ministrations. The dispensary was the place where they could find expert treatment, even if often casual and in undignified surroundings.

With such an enormous amount of institutional practice it was inevitable that many ordinary clinicians should have come to resent the free care provided by "hospital doctors"—which they saw as a factor in reducing their already meager incomes. A good proportion of dispensary patients, they argued, could perfectly well pay for private care, but chose instead to present themselves as indigent so as to benefit from and take advantage of these gratuitous services. Hospital staffers were resented as complicit in perpetuating such "dispensary abuse," motivated by their selfish desire for "teaching material." Despite such criticisms, dispensaries and hospital services generally expanded rapidly at the end of the nineteenth century.

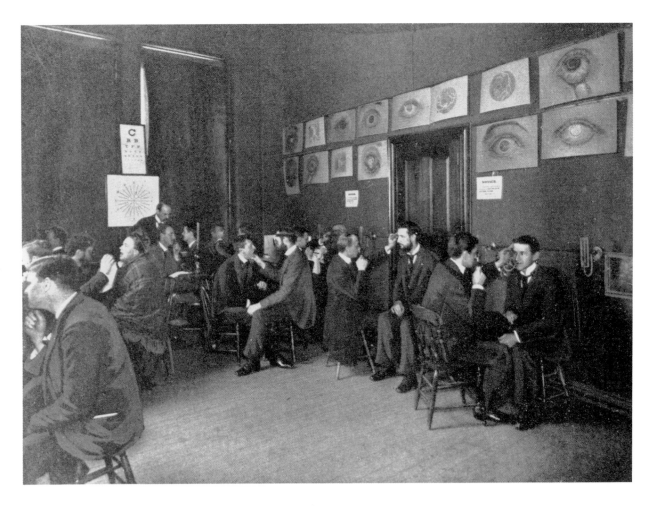

45.

Eye clinic, Hahnemann
Hospital.
*Archives, Hahnemann
University.*

HOSPITAL CLINICS SOON became the center for specialty care and clinical training, and ophthalmology was one of the earliest medical specialties.
Here, physicians in the eye clinic at Hahnemann
Hospital in 1890 are busy practicing their diagnostic skills.

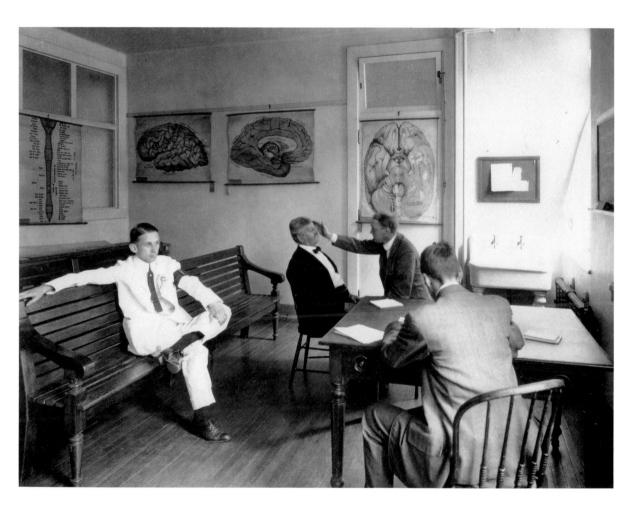

THE CREATION OF neurology as a medical specialty organized around a somatic view of behavioral "pathology" occurred in the second half of the nineteenth century. As was the case with many other specialties, neurology found its first general hospital foothold in outpatient departments. In this photograph, a patient is undergoing an examination in the nervous dispensary of the Hospital of the University of Pennsylvania in 1911.

46.

Nervous dispensary, Hospital of the University of Pennsylvania.
University of Pennsylvania Archives.

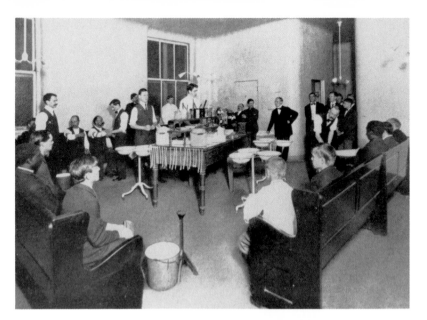

IN CROWDED DISPENSARIES in the late nineteenth and early twentieth centuries there was little or no privacy; treatment was provided in a public area, easily visible to those waiting their turn. The creation of the curtained treatment area and later the private consultation room must be considered as reflecting changing views of class and sensibility—as well as the recruitment of a more varied patient population.

The public nature of the outpatient dispensary can be seen in these images of an adult surgical clinic at Thomas Jefferson University Hospital and a surgical dispensary at the Children's Hospital of Philadelphia.

47.

Surgical clinic, Jefferson Hospital.
Thomas Jefferson University, Scott Memorial Library.

48.

Surgical dispensary, Children's Hospital of Philadelphia.
Children's Hospital of Philadelphia.

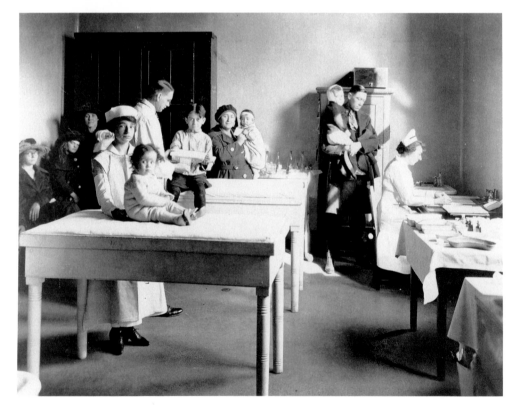

THE ENTRANCE OF middle-class women and men into the hospital encouraged a growing respect for patient privacy. This notion of privacy emerged only gradually in wards and clinics. Taken in 1931, this photograph of the consultation area at the medical dispensary of Hahnemann Hospital displays how treatment areas could be separated by curtains. Finally, in an image familiar to modern clinic visitors, we can see an outpatient waiting room, organized so that patients could anticipate consultations in largely private surroundings. This 1945 photograph was taken at the Hospital of the University of Pennsylvania.

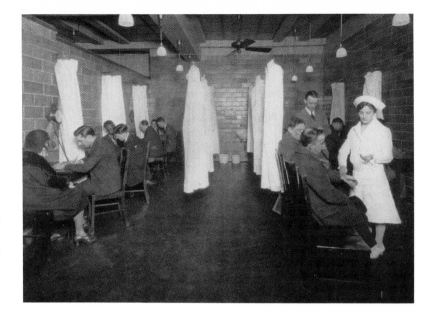

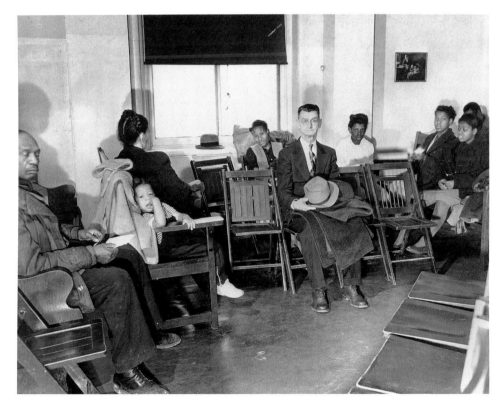

49.

Medical dispensary, Hahnemann Hospital. *Archives, Hahnemann University.*

50.

Outpatient waiting room, Hospital of the University of Pennsylvania. *University of Pennsylvania Archives.*

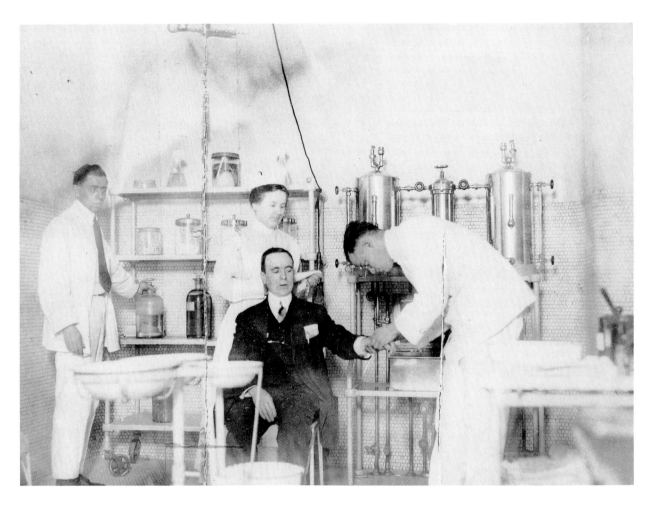

51.

Emergency room, Jefferson Hospital.
Thomas Jefferson University, Scott Memorial Library.

ONE PATH TO the ward or private bed began in the emergency room, where accident cases were treated. Until the twentieth century, middle-class accident victims were often taken from the scene to their homes where they could be attended by their private physicians. But by World War I the hospital had become the expected and appropriate site of emergency care. Patients assumed that hospitals should provide a specialized emergency function, one capable of dealing promptly and effectively with trauma and other medical emergencies. This emergency room at Thomas Jefferson University Hospital in 1916 reassures through the presence of a gleaming technical capacity.

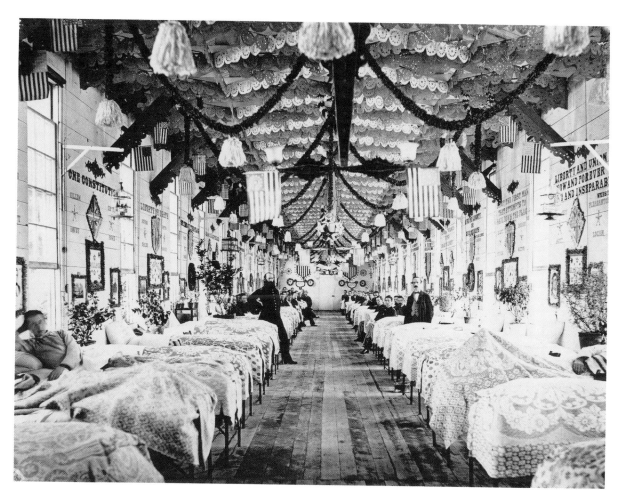

THE WARD CONSTITUTED one of the late-nineteenth- and early-twentieth-century hospital's most enduring aspects. Most were simply large rectangular rooms with beds jutting from each wall. This configuration with its standard ventilation and heating arrangements was often termed a "Nightingale Ward" after English nursing reformer Florence Nightingale (1820–1910), whose writings on hospital design and management were so influential during the second half of the nineteenth century. Thus this photograph from the Nicetown Civil War Hospital in 1862 seems almost jarring with its luxurious decorations: lace bedspreads, flags, streamers, and posters honor the wounded Union soldiers filling its beds. But even with such atypical embellishment, it is instantly recognizable as a hospital ward.

52.

Nicetown Civil War Hospital ward.
The Library Company of Philadelphia.

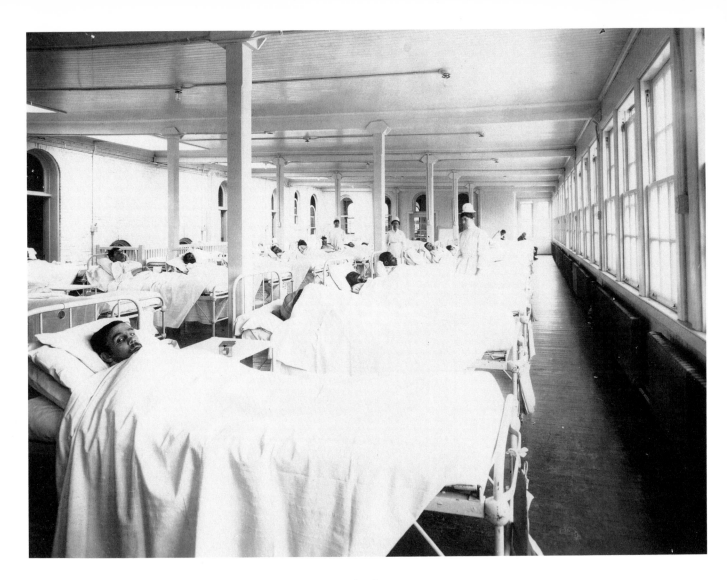

53.

Tubercular men's ward, Philadelphia General Hospital.
Historical Collections, College of Physicians of Philadelphia.

SEX AND DIAGNOSIS typically determined a patient's ward assignment in large hospitals. There were wards for medical and surgical cases, and wards organized along clinical specialty lines were sometimes established in general hospitals along with wards for contagious diseases. The first image shows men with tuberculosis at the Philadelphia General Hospital. The second is a women's ward at the Hospital of the University of Pennsylvania in the 1940s.

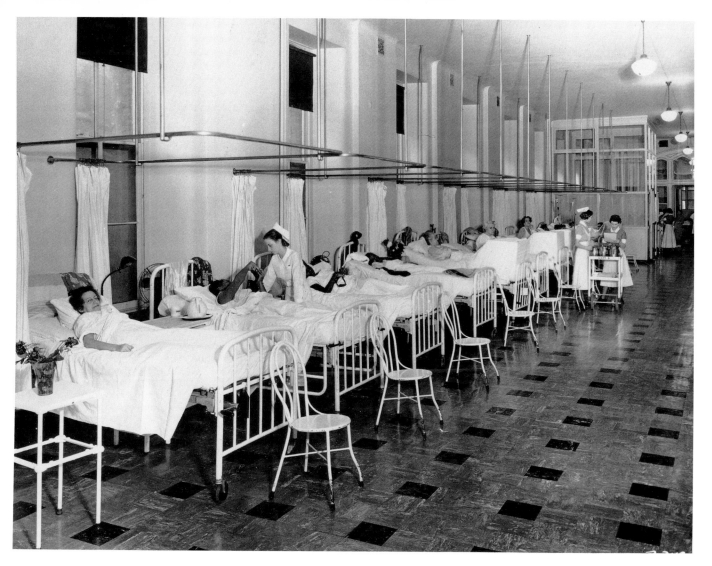

54.

Women's ward, Hospital
of the University of
Pennsylvania.
*University of Pennsyl-
vania Archives.*

CHILDBIRTH MOVED FROM home to hospital during the twentieth century. Initially only poor women, unable to afford a physician or midwife—and sometimes even a clean bed and regular meals—gave birth in the hospital. Until the late 1930s hospital births, which involved occasional surgical intervention and the possible use of drugs and instruments, were no safer and possibly more dangerous than home births. Nevertheless, hospitals attracted increasing numbers of women, in part because of the availability of anesthesia, offering the promise of "painless childbirth." By 1940, 55 percent of all births took place in the hospital.

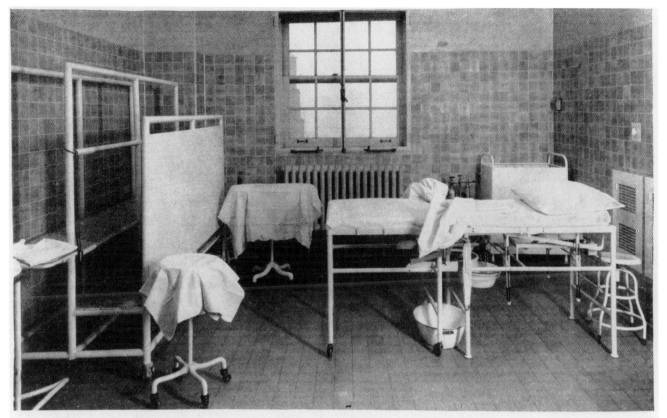

Every facility of modern obstetrical and gynecological science is available for the new mother and her baby

AT THE END of the twentieth century we have become accustomed to hospitals promoting their "homelike" delivery rooms. In the 1930s, when hospitals sought to encourage middle-class women to use their private and semi-private services, their advertising highlighted the sterile and scientifically well-equipped delivery room. There is nothing homelike in *this* Pennsylvania Hospital delivery room. As the original caption indicates, hospitals sought to use photographs to communicate a reassuring sense of science and efficiency.

55.

Delivery room, Pennsylvania Hospital.
Pennsylvania Hospital Archives.

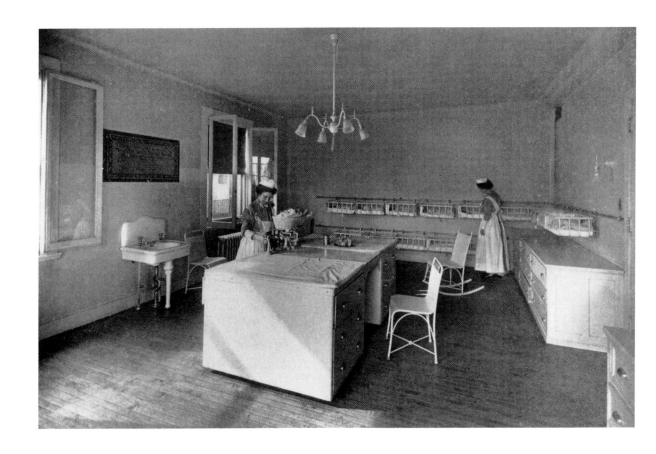

56.

Nursery with wall cribs,
Hahnemann Hospital.
*Archives, Hahnemann
University.*

WITH THEIR ROWS of babies in bassinets and
presiding nurses in well-starched uniforms, nurseries, like surgical amphitheaters, were often
photographed. Typical of these images was the
nursery at Hahnemann Hospital, with its wall
cribs, photographed in 1908, and the nursery sun-
parlor at Thomas Jefferson University Hospital
from the 1920s.

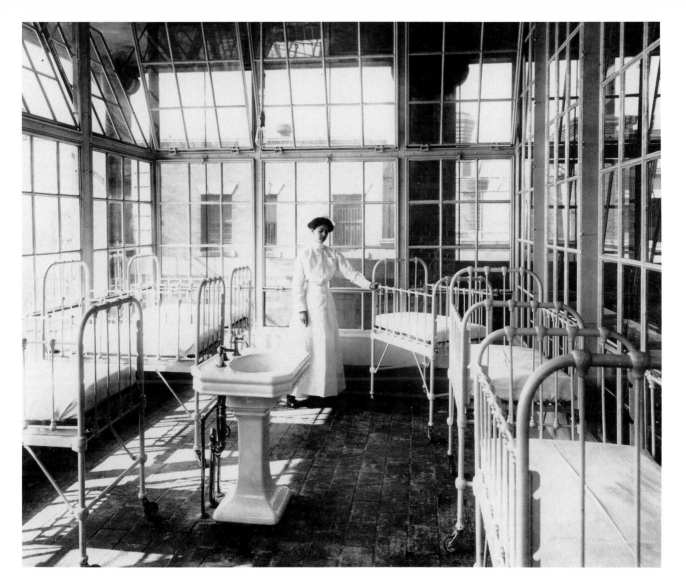

57.

Nursery sun-parlor,
Jefferson Hospital.
*Thomas Jefferson Univer-
sity, Scott Memorial
Library.*

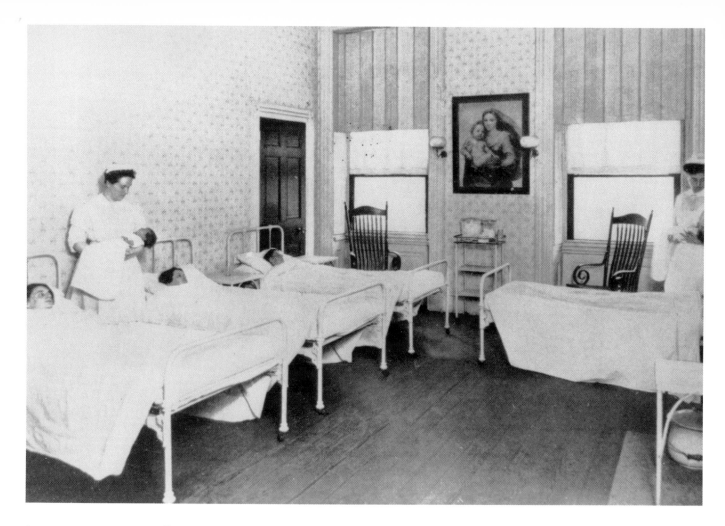

58.

Maternity ward, Jefferson Hospital.
Thomas Jefferson University, Scott Memorial Library.

FOR IMPOVERISHED URBAN women in the late nineteenth and early twentieth centuries, a hospital birth was often the only choice. Unable to afford a midwife, lacking the help and amenities for home confinement, they gave birth in a hospital bed. House officers and senior medical students managed the deliveries, and in complicated cases experienced practitioners were available to assist them. After delivery the women usually remained in the institution for several weeks in maternity wards such as this one, photographed at Jefferson Hospital in 1907.

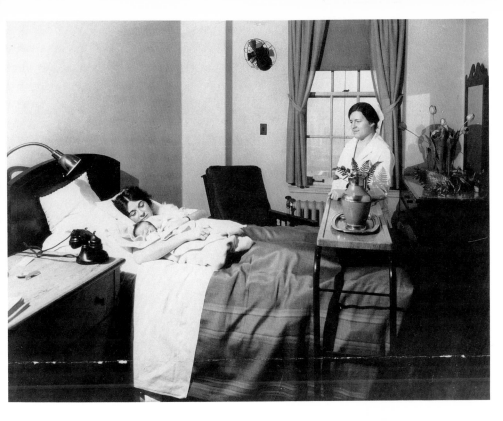

59.

Private maternity bed, Pennsylvania Hospital. *Pennsylvania Hospital Archives.*

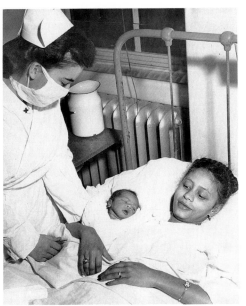

60.

Maternity ward bed. *Charles L. Blockson Afro-American Collection, Temple University.*

THE MOVEMENT OF birth into the hospital in the first half of the twentieth century reflected a number of factors. Significant among them was the attraction of anesthesia and the perception that hospital birth was safer than home birth for mothers and babies. Photographers captured this transition in formulaic images of new mothers and babies cared for by attentive hospital nurses. An obviously posed image advertises the comforts of a private room at the Pennsylvania Hospital in 1930. But there are many similar elements in the photograph of a hospital ward bed, circa 1940.

THE DEVELOPMENT OF the modern general hospital in the late nineteenth and early twentieth centuries coincided with the emergence of pediatrics as a medical specialty. In general hospitals children began to be cared for in separate wards and in many cities children's hospitals were erected. Philadelphians founded a number of institutions for children, including the Children's Hospital of Philadelphia, opened in 1855 (the first such hospital in the United States), St. Christopher's Hospital for Children, established in 1875, the Children's Homeopathic Hospital of Philadelphia, founded in 1877, and the Babies Hospital, which opened its doors in 1911. Like their counterparts for adults, these institutions initially served the poor and especially the victims of chronic and orthopedic ailments; they evolved slowly into modern acute-care facilities serving patients of all classes.

Even as developments in scientific medicine reshaped their technical capacities, the legacy of social welfare continued to influence both the public role and the internal operations of children's wards and hospitals. Specially trained nurses and social workers helped to ensure that medical care was supplied in a manner befitting the special social needs of children. Unlike the often drab and cheerless adult wards, children's wards were often well appointed. And unlike the distanced and self-conscious professional demeanors of the staff common to photographs taken on adult wards, these photographs show physicians and nurses seemingly moved by the plight of their young patients.

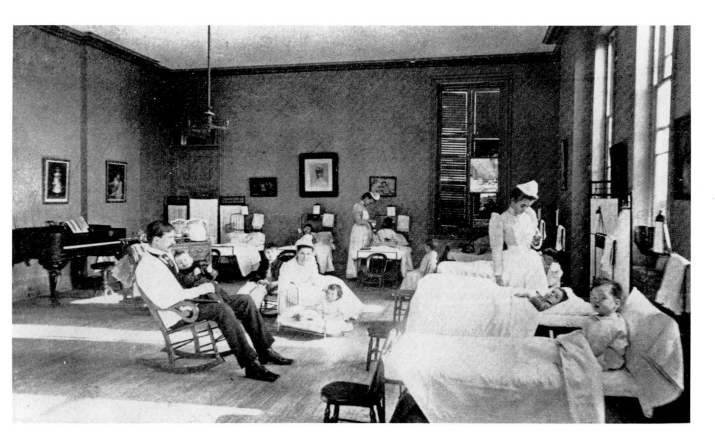

THE CAPTIVATING FACES of children and the poi-
gnancy of their condition drew generations of
photographers to the children's wards. What these
images collectively reveal is the degree to which
children were given special treatment, not so
much in terms of medical techniques but in regard
to their social identity. The first image, taken on
the girls' surgical ward of the Children's Hospital
of Philadelphia in 1892, illustrates the adminis-
tration's effort to make the accommodations comfortable for its young patients. The walls are decorated with pictures and a piano is present.

61.

Girls' surgical ward,
Children's Hospital of
Philadelphia.
*Children's Hospital of
Philadelphia.*

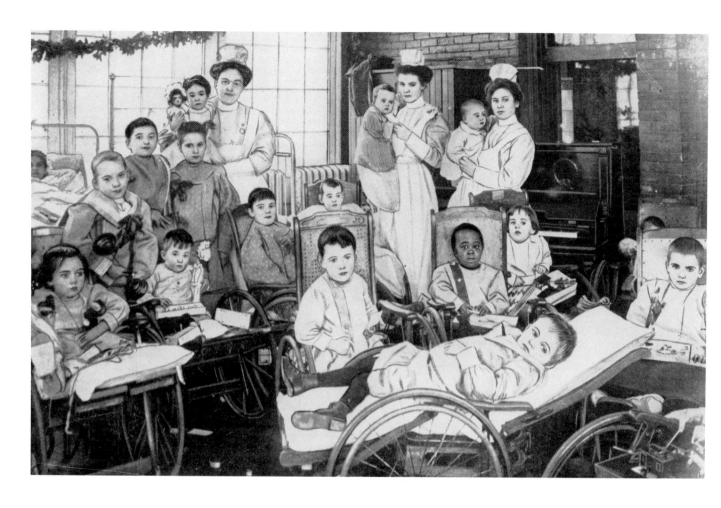

62.

Pediatric ward, Hospital
of the University of
Pennsylvania.
*Historical Collections,
College of Physicians of
Philadelphia.*

A PIANO CAN also be seen in this retouched 1910
image from the Hospital of the University of
Pennsylvania; its sentimental original caption
reads "Little Patients After Kris Kringle's Visit."
As the wheelchairs in this image suggest, a significant portion of pediatric inpatients suffered
from orthopedic problems.

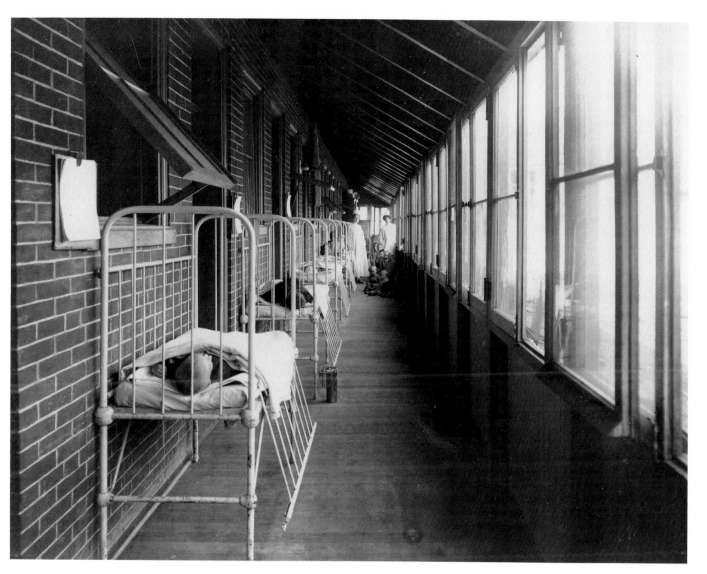

ACUTE, CONTAGIOUS DISEASES of childhood also brought many young patients to the hospital. And in the era before preventive inoculations there were an abundance of such sufferers. Before effective antibiotic therapy and other modern therapeutic modalities the hospital could only supply good nursing, a clean environment, rest, healthy food, and sunshine. A 1910 photograph from the whooping cough ward of the Philadelphia General Hospital illustrates the provision of "fresh air and sunshine."

63.

Whooping cough ward, Philadelphia General Hospital.
City Archives of Philadelphia.

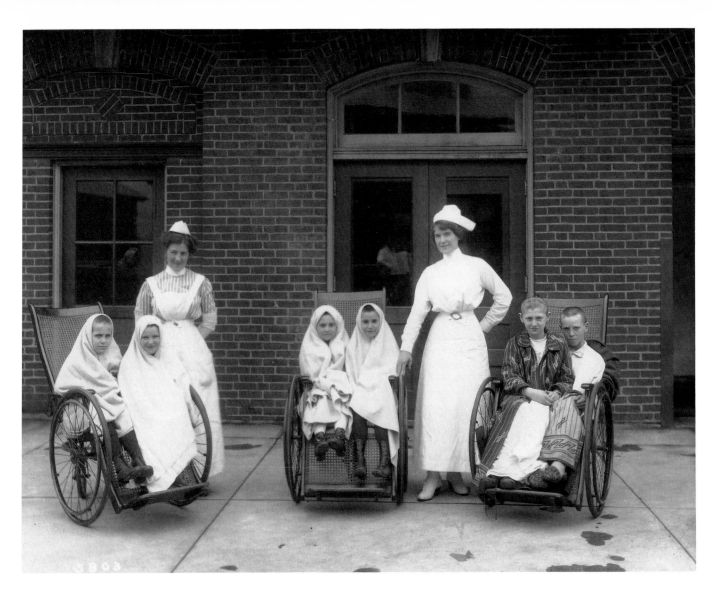

64.

Children receiving sunshine therapy.
City Archives of Philadelphia.

UNTIL THE TWENTIETH century, hospital care consisted in general not in intrusive treatment for a specific illness, but in provision of a nourishing diet, warmth, rest, and attentive nursing. Hospitals facilitated, but could not accelerate, the healing power of nature; most ills followed their natural course to recovery or death. Patients remained hospitalized or in convalescent facilities until they regained strength and vigor. For those with cer-

tain chronic ailments, sunshine therapy was considered indispensable. Thus many photographs of both adult and children's wards show patients at rest on a sun porch. In this 1912 photograph young convalescents are enjoying "a sun bake."

PRIVATE-ROOM INCOME became increasingly important to hospitals, and well-to-do patients were lured to the hospital with the promise of luxurious accommodations, fine food, and extensive visiting hours. Unlike the ward patients, whose admission was sometimes preceded by a bath and a delousing and whose stay was punctuated by the prying eyes, hands, and instruments of medical students, private-room patients were guaranteed a good measure of privacy. This respect was assured by the photographer as well. Ward patients were often before the camera's eye; private rooms were usually photographed empty. Thus this first image, taken at Hahnemann Hospital in 1893, is unusual, while the second from the Hospital of the University of Pennsylvania in 1910 is more typical.

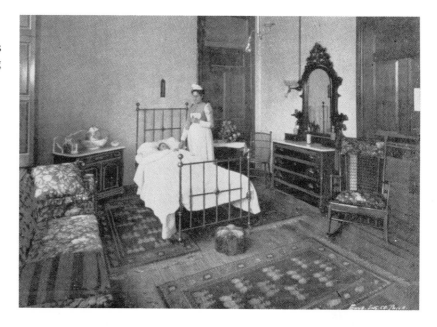

65.

Private room, Hahnemann Hospital.
Archives, Hahnemann University.

66.

Private room, Hospital of the University of Pennsylvania.
Historical Collections, College of Physicians of Philadelphia.

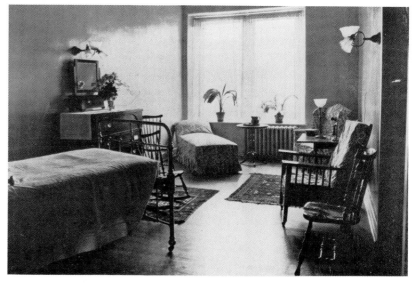

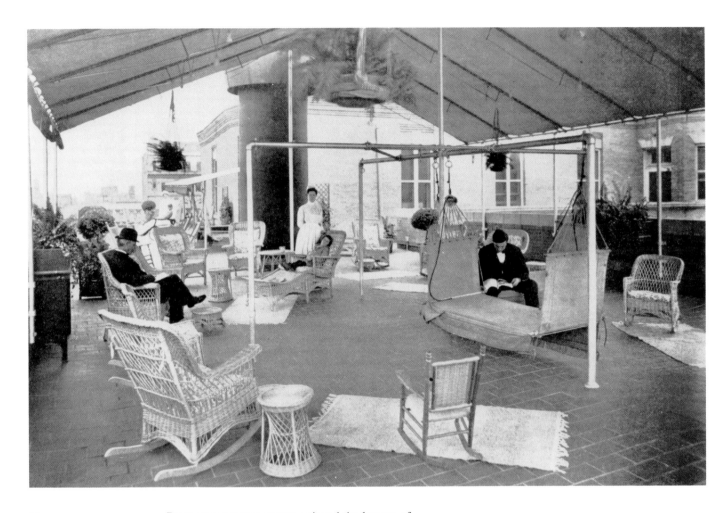

67.

Sun porch, Jefferson
Hospital.
*Historical Collections,
College of Physicians of
Philadelphia.*

PRIVATE PATIENTS OFTEN enjoyed the luxury of
a private roof garden, such as this one at the
Jefferson Medical College (now Thomas Jefferson
University) Hospital as photographed in 1915.

THE ROOTS OF the American hospital are to be found in the almshouse, in
the experience of poverty as much as that of illness. As early as 1732 the
Philadelphia Almshouse designated an infirmary for the sick and insane, and
through the early nineteenth century wards were set aside for those too ill to
work. By 1826, for example, thirteen of eighteen women's wards were filled
with medical patients. Similarly, fifteen of nineteen men's wards housed the
sick. Differentiating between disease and dependency was, in fact, no easy
matter; the elderly might be housed on sick wards when beds were available,
and moved to outwards (for indigent, healthy inmates) when the sick wards
became too crowded. Dependency rather than diagnosis was the primary
factor shaping admission.

The creation of a formal municipal hospital awaited the relocation of the
almshouse from the city's downtown to a more distant site in Blockley town-
ship—now West Philadelphia. By 1833 patients began to be transferred to
the new site. Officially designated the Philadelphia Hospital, and renamed
Philadelphia General Hospital in 1902, the institution was always referred to
as Blockley. At the end of the nineteenth century it comprised a sprawling
variety of structures including a maternity pavilion, older wooden and newer
brick pavilions for medical patients, apartments for nurses, laboratories, a
children's hospital, special buildings for the insane and the tubercular, an
isolation unit for the contagious, and other buildings such as the electric
plant and pathological museum. Blockley's physical differentiation mirrored
both the breadth of Philadelphia's medical and social problems and the increasing subdivision of medicine into areas of specialization.

The physicians and nurses who trained at Blockley contended with dependency and sickness on a large scale. The patient census in 1887, for
example, was 1,200—while the Pennsylvania Hospital was treating a mere
164 men and women. Furthermore, Blockley patients entered the hospital
only as a last resort; to be treated in the "almshouse hospital" was to be
burdened with the stigma of pauperism. Some were admitted when turned
away at voluntary hospitals. Others were referred directly by "outdoor physicians" paid by the city to care for the sick and indigent in their homes.
Entering through Blockley's gates were a variety of patients unwelcome at
any of the city's numerous charity hospitals: the chronically ill, the tubercular, the alcoholic, and the moribund.

While the combination of poverty and sickness continued to bring numerous patients to Blockley, a growing medicalization led to the separation of
some kinds of patients. In the late nineteenth century, for example, organic
neurological ills and epilepsy cases were transferred from the hospital's

"mental wards." (Blockley's chronic neurological wards, with their difficult patients scorned by other hospitals, soon became a center for teaching and clinical investigation.) Other categories of patients were also shifted to new treatment sites. "Feeble-minded" children were sent to the training school at Elwyn, those best categorized as the "vagrant and semi-criminal class" were dispatched to the House of Correction, and, finally, in the twentieth century, the chronically insane were sent to the hospital erected at Byberry and the well poor moved to the Home for the Indigent in Holmesburg.

68.

Bird's eye view, Philadelphia General Hospital. *Center for the Study of the History of Nursing, School of Nursing, University of Pennsylvania.*

69.

Ward plan, Philadelphia General Hospital. *City Archives of Philadelphia.*

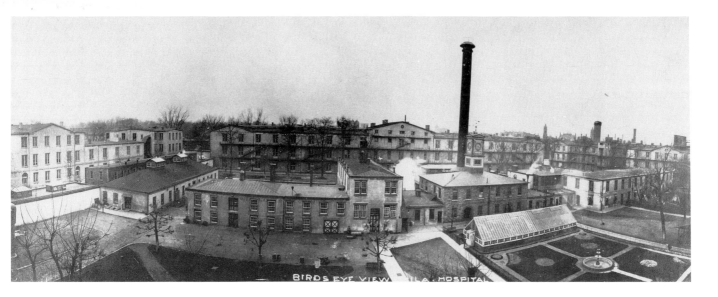

BIRDS EYE VIEW PHILA. HOSPITAL

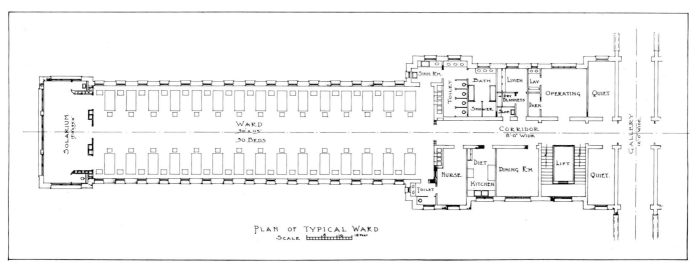

PLAN OF TYPICAL WARD
SCALE _____ 16 FEET

THE REMOVAL OF the mentally ill and others did little to deplete the supply of patients. Until its closing in 1977, Philadelphia General Hospital remained a large-scale enterprise in terms of patient census and professional activity. In this bird's eye view of its buildings and grounds Blockley resembles a nineteenth-century industrial worksite, a sprawling medical factory. This architectural plan of a typical ward, containing thirty beds, possibly from the 1906 renovations of the male outwards, gives another suggestion of the scale of the institution.

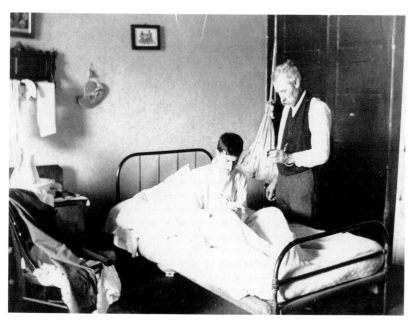

Some Blockley physicians recorded their experiences in diaries and reminiscences, while others used a camera. John L. Bower (1865–1955), a resident in 1888, George E. Pfahler (1874–1957), a resident in 1898, and Robert J. Hunter (1882–1980), a resident between 1904 and 1906, were among those who photographed their Blockley days. Bower's views from 1888 include two reproduced here: a young house officer, Dr. Milton Rosenau, responding to a note brought by a night messenger from a patient and a House of Correction gang brought to Blockley to do laboring work. The image of the bread wagon delivering loaves from the hospital's central bakery was taken by Dr. Pfahler about 1900. Together the images suggest the range of activity within this complex institution.

70.

Physician responding to message from patient, Philadelphia General Hospital.
Historical Collections, College of Physicians of Philadelphia.

71.

House of Correction gang at Philadelphia General Hospital.
Historical Collections, College of Physicians of Philadelphia.

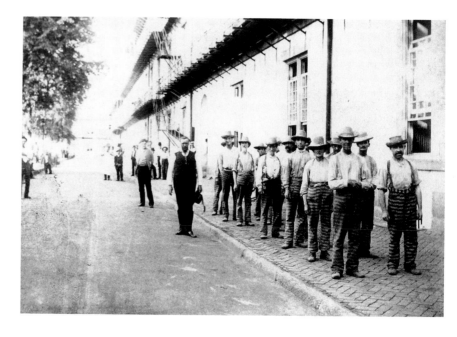

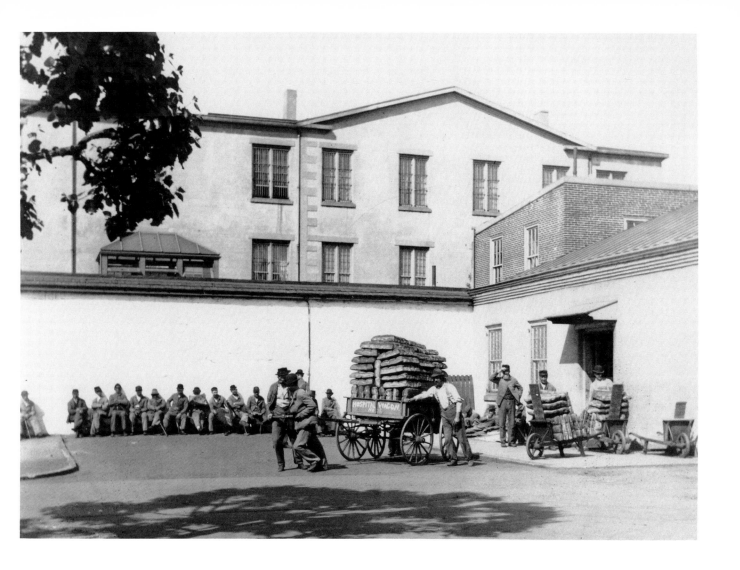

72.

Bread truck, Philadelphia
General Hospital.
*Historical Collections,
College of Physicians of
Philadelphia.*

73.

Children outside outward, Philadelphia General Hospital.
Center for the Study of the History of Nursing, School of Nursing, University of Pennsylvania.

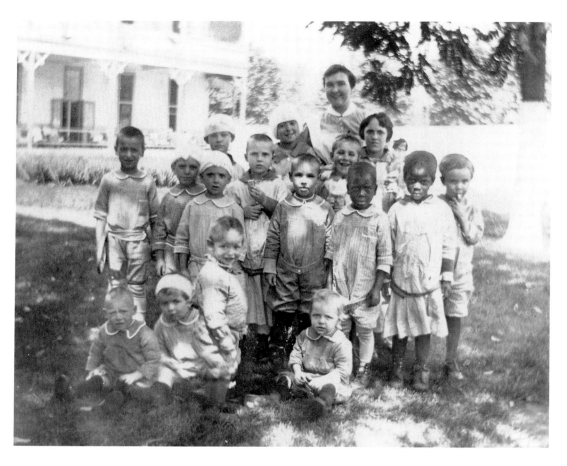

WHILE WE HAVE come to think of hospitals as places in which patients were confined indoors, images of Philadelphia General Hospital often suggest the contrary. For those able or required to be up and about the immense grounds were well used. Here children are posing outside their wooden ward. They are wearing institutional clothing and some have had their heads shaved and wrapped as treatment for lice infestations. Many of those treated in the children's asylum were orphans or chronic cases who could not be placed elsewhere. In the words of one visitor, they were "deformed, crippled, diseased eyes, nervous, etc." The question of whether they were the responsibility of welfare or medicine was moot; they had nowhere else to go.

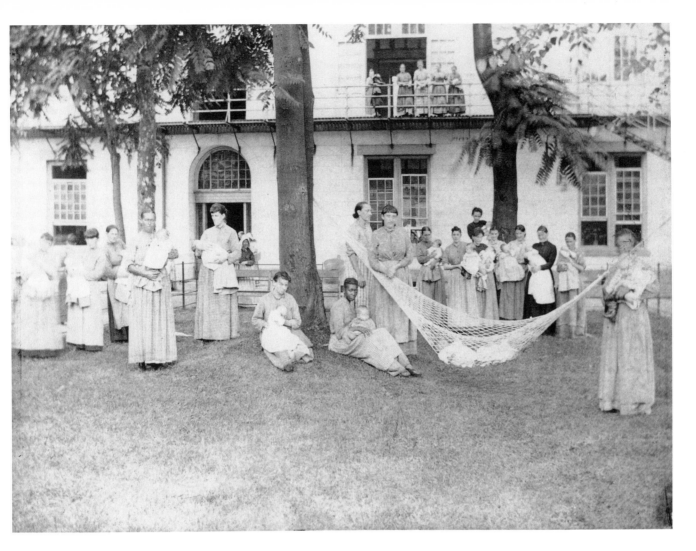

MATERNITY CASES, SHOWN here at the turn of the century, also occupied a gray area between the domains of medicine and welfare. In 1883, when the maternity pavilion was established, the obstetric staff recommended restricting patient stays to three months after confinement, but undoubtedly many lingered longer, having no other place to go and no means of support. Before the twentieth century no respectable middle-class woman would have consented to give birth in a hospital bed.

Dr. Arthur Ames Bliss (1859–1913), describing his service in 1883–1884, wrote: "We had no case of puerperal fever during our term. Yet this was partly a coincidence or good luck; for the walls, floors and furniture of those old rooms must have been loaded with streptococci, staphylococci, pneumococci, and all the noble army of the bacillus gens."

74.

Maternity pavilion, Philadelphia General Hospital. *Historical Collections, College of Physicians of Philadelphia.*

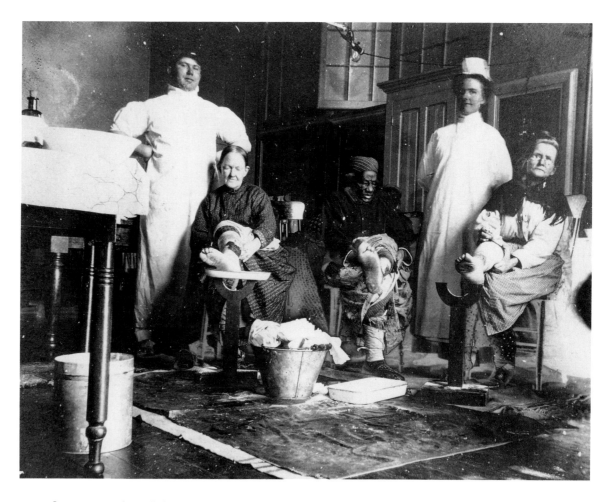

75.

Leg ulcer clinic, Phila-
delphia General Hospital.
*Historical Collections,
College of Physicians of
Philadelphia.*

IN THE LEG ulcer clinic, shown here in 1904,
Dr. Walter Bowers (1855–1947) stands ready to
treat his patients. Leg ulcers, as the photograph
suggests, were more common among women
than men.

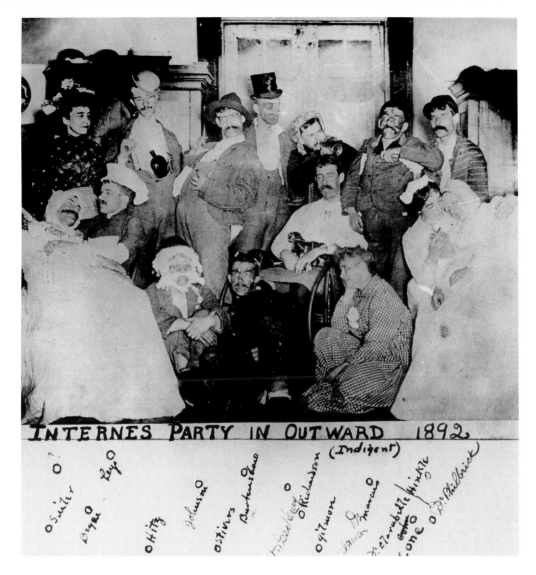

INTERNES PARTY IN OUTWARD 1892.
(Indigent)

76.

Interns' party in outward,
Philadelphia General
Hospital.
*Historical Collections,
College of Physicians of
Philadelphia.*

NOT ONLY WERE patients sick and needy, they could be dangerous. A physician, one resident warned, "must be wary, if he wants to have control of his wards, for the vicious and often criminal elements therein will stop short of nothing to circumvent him." The social distance between physicians and patients was ordinarily unbridgeable, and one resident confessed that "After living in such circumstances, we became naturally overbearing, dogmatic, and it must be confessed more or less brutal." It is not surprising then that physician-photographers sometimes staged scenes that mocked and ridiculed the patients. In this one, labeled by its creator "Internes Party in Outward, (Indigent) 1892," physicians have donned patients' clothing and seem to be caricaturing the "inmates" and hospital staff.

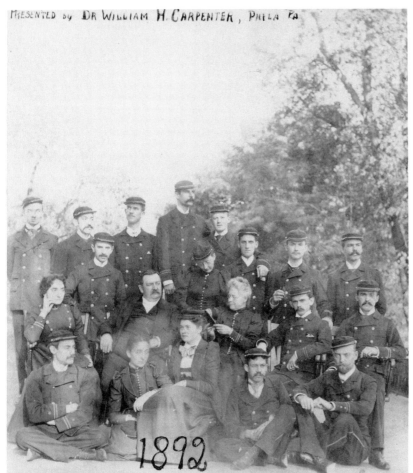

PRESENTED BY DR. WILLIAM H. CARPENTER, PHILA PA

1892

TOP ROW — TRUMAN AUGÉ, HERMAN D. MARCUS, CHAS. C. STIVERS,
WM. MARSHALL HINKLE, JAMES H. McKEE, ALVAH M. DAVIS,
WILLIAM H. CARPENTER, SIDNEY MONTEGUT
MIDDLE ROW — CLARIBEL CONE, DAVID RIESMAN.
CHIEF DANIEL E. HUGHES, INEZ C. PHILBRICK, AMELIA
W GILMORE, WM. E BRUNER, GLENDON E. CURRY.
BOTTOM ROW — JOSEPH SAILER, FLORA POLLACK,
MARY GREENWALD ERDMAN, HENRY D. BEYEA, J.H.BURTENSHAW

DESPITE THE DIFFICULTIES of working at Block-ley, it provided excellent clinical training. One former resident commented that "Blockley is an unhealthy, miserable place to live, but it is very healthy for growth in medical knowledge." In 1890, *Philadelphia Hospital Reports* was begun as a vehicle for the publication of clinical studies conducted at Blockley; in 1904, the hospital's annual report included a bibliography of articles in which Blockley "materials" had been used. Slowly the former almshouse was integrated into the modern world of medicine and medical research. The experience of house officership became an increasingly significant aspect of the American practitioner's training; it was a grueling task, yet inspired pride and confidence.

The same group who posed as mock patients are shown here in their uniforms (copied from the uniforms of navy surgeons) as the residents' class of 1892. The uniforms represent one aspect of a more comprehensive effort to impose a bureaucratic order on what had been an unruly working-class institution; the professionalization of Blockley nursing—begun in 1885—constituted a particularly important aspect of such ordered change.

77.

Blockley interns in uniform.
Historical Collections, College of Physicians of Philadelphia.

ADVANCES IN DIAGNOSIS and treatment helped transform the general hospital from a welfare to a seemingly medical institution; for the mentally ill there were no such breakthroughs. While an increased understanding of the behavioral manifestations of mental illness allowed for more sophisticated classification of patients and in some conditions, such as syphilis and pellagra, preventive or therapeutic management of somatic complaints, the prognosis for the great majority—in the twentieth century as in the late nineteenth—was poor.

The shifting of certain categories of patients, such as alcoholics and the elderly senile, to other facilities also helped to change the patient census at Philadelphia's mental hospitals. The discovery of effective anti-syphilitic and anti-epileptic drugs also removed some patients. Those who remained behind suffered in most instances from chronic and intractable complaints. A variety of treatments were used, including occupational therapy, sedatives, hydrotherapy, and in the 1920s and 1930s insulin and metrozal shock. In the 1940s and 1950s psycho-surgery enjoyed a vogue; the allure of an effective somatic intervention remained powerful so long as difficult chronic patients filled hospital beds.

Perhaps no other category of health care displays so vividly the differences in treatment provided to the rich and the poor. Images of private mental hospitals, well furnished, well staffed, and well maintained, contrast sharply with the large overburdened public institutions suffering from overcrowding and a lack of funds. Moreover, while private patients were rarely photographed, a reflection of the stigma surrounding mental illness, the life of the mentally ill in public institutions is rather well documented. Although private general hospital patients were also spared the photographer's intrusions, the distance between the private room and the general hospital ward was not as great as that between the private and the public mental hospital.

PRIVATE MENTAL HOSPITALS

CHARITABLE PHILADELPHIANS WERE pioneers in American efforts to provide institutional care for the mentally ill. The Pennsylvania Hospital treated such patients from its opening in 1752. It soon developed a reputation for the management of these vexing cases and began to attract private patients from outside the state. In 1817 the Friends' Asylum opened its doors, founded with the intent of providing humane care to Friends "bereft of their reason."

By the 1820s Pennsylvania Hospital found the numbers of insane and the difficulty of treating them in a general hospital overwhelming. They sought a separate site for their "lunatic patients" and found a rural area some miles west; in 1841 the Insane Department of the Pennsylvania Hospital (now the Institute of Pennsylvania Hospital) opened. Under the leadership of Thomas Story Kirkbride—superintendent between 1840 and 1883—it soon became a leader in the private hospital care of the mentally ill.

Private hospitals admitted small numbers of patients. The average daily patient census at Friends Hospital in 1935 was 128, while at the Institute of Pennsylvania Hospital it was 173. At some of the smaller, private facilities, such as the Kenwood Sanitarium, the number was even lower, only 29. By contrast, the daily average at the public hospital, the Philadelphia Hospital for Mental Diseases (Byberry), was 5,634.

Photographs of comfortable private rooms devoid of patients helped market both private accommodations in general hospitals and private mental hospitals. This image of a bedroom and sitting room at Friends Hospital in 1922 is reminiscent of those taken of private rooms in general hospitals. Friends Hospital has remained a private mental hospital, located in the city's Northeast area.

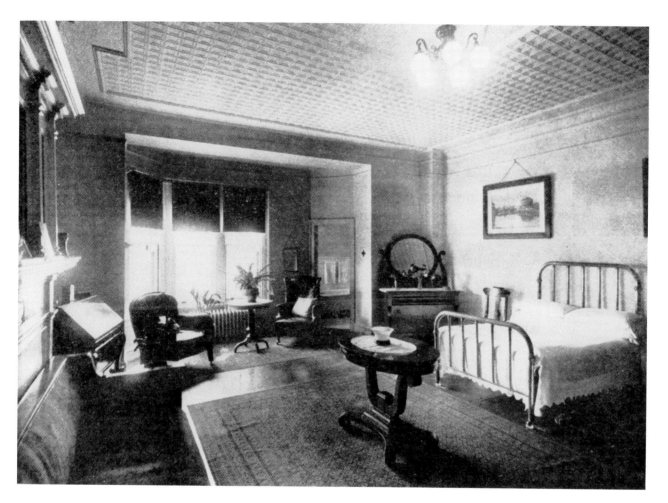

78.

Private room, Friends
Hospital.
*Historical Collections,
College of Physicians of
Philadelphia.*

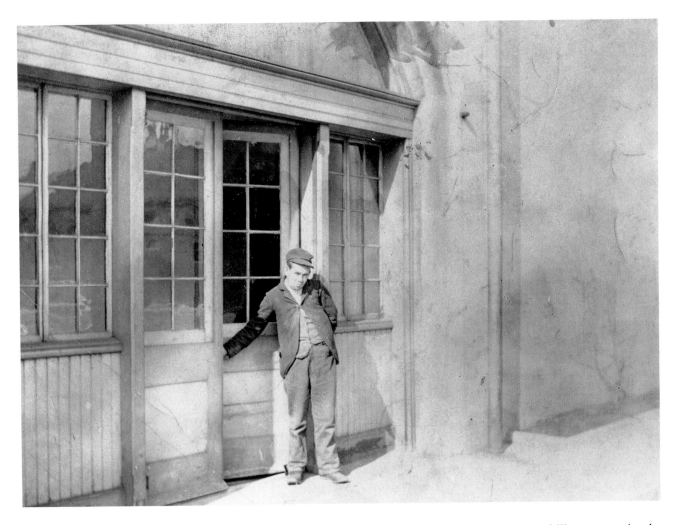

79.

Pete Malone, Philadelphia General Hospital.
Center for the Study of the History of Nursing, School of Nursing, University of Pennsylvania.

UNTIL THE OPENING of the Philadelphia Hospital for Mental Diseases, known as Byberry, Philadelphia General Hospital housed thousands of insane patients who had been legally committed to its care. Among them was Pete Malone, shown here opening the doors to the men's nervous ward. In the second image, female patients from the insane department pose in the yard. The wards for patients suffering from mental illnesses consisted of long wooden pavilions, recalled by one resident as "hardly better than shacks."

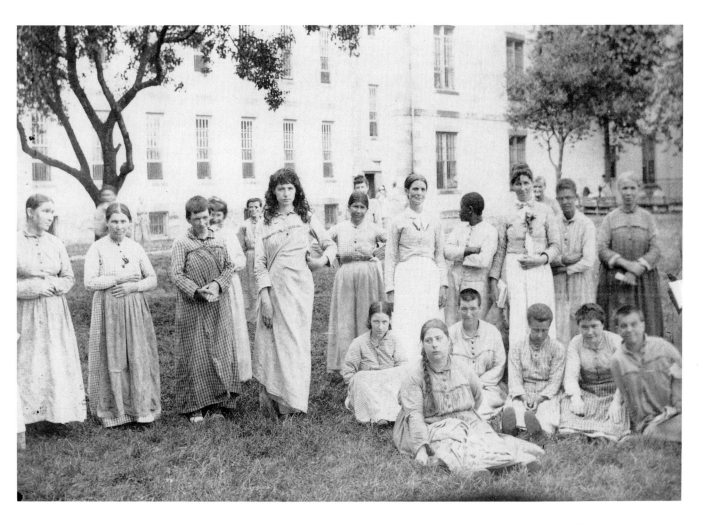

80.

Insane female patients,
Philadelphia General
Hospital.
*Historical Collections,
College of Physicians of
Philadelphia.*

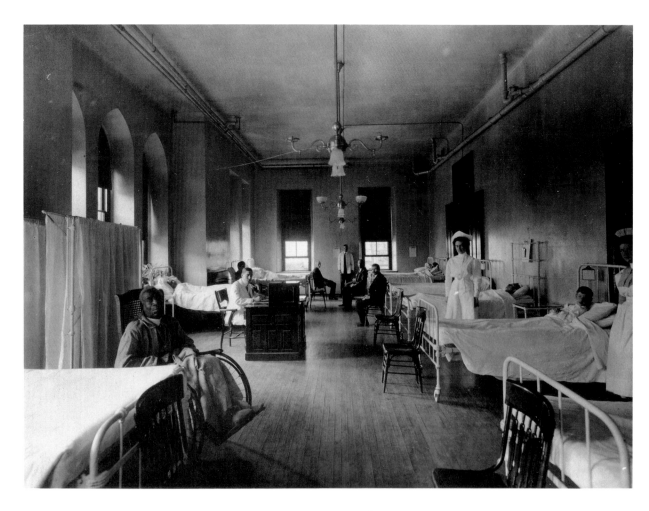

81.

Men's nervous ward, Hospital of the University of Pennsylvania.
University of Pennsylvania Archives.

IN THE FIRST decades of the twentieth century, many urban teaching hospitals created neurological and acute psychiatric services. The Hospital of the University of Pennsylvania too followed this self-consciously enlightened policy.

The mix of patients in the men's nervous ward at the Hospital of the University of Pennsylvania in 1911 is striking. On the left there is an elderly man confined to a wheelchair, on the right a young boy confined to bed. The photograph seems obviously staged, with its nurses, patients, and physician seated at a desk and all staring at the camera.

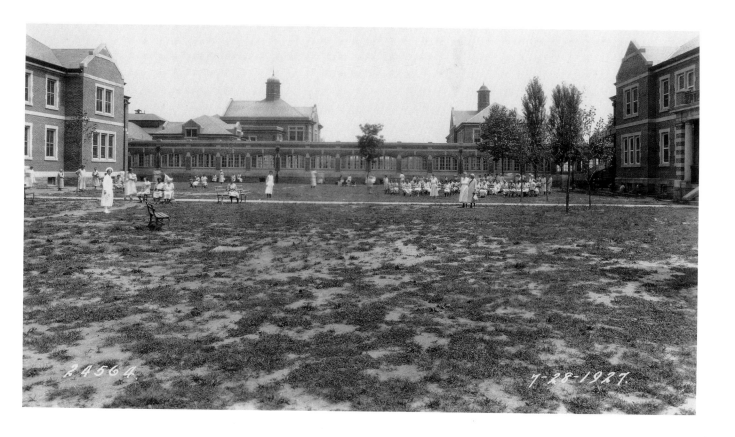

24564   7-28-1927

REFORMERS CALLED FOR the establishment of a separate, specialized facility to be used in treating the mentally ill, and in 1926, 1,400 Blockley patients diagnosed as insane were moved to a bucolic setting northeast of central Philadelphia. The distance allowed it to maintain a working farm, but also made the institution less visible. As was the case in many secluded and largely chronic mental hospitals, custodial care on a lim-ited budget created dismal conditions and became a source of recurring exposés and scandals.

Byberry, like its sister hospital, Blockley, was a rambling, multistructured, and crowded institu-tion. This official 1927 photograph of the female yard and surrounding buildings is suggestive of a college campus. In a more revealing photograph taken that same year (see next page), the chil-dren's dining room resembles a reformatory.

82.

Exterior view of Byberry.
City Archives of Philadelphia.

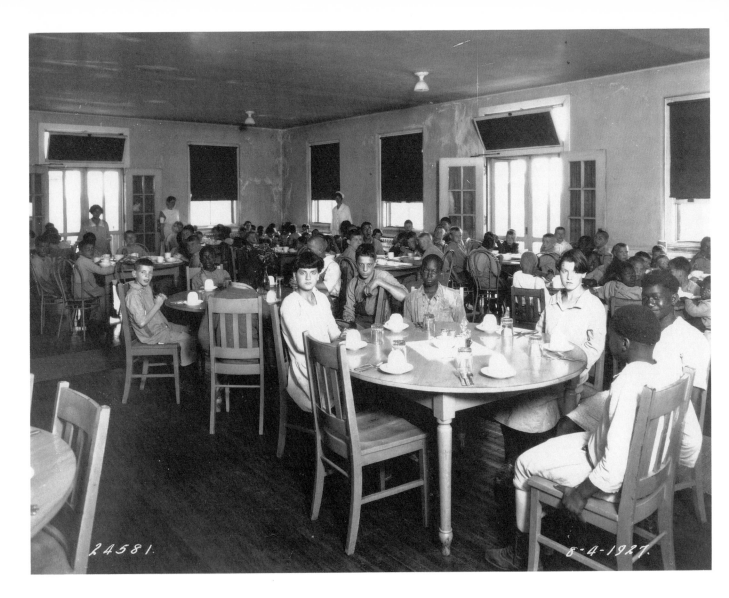

83.

Children's dining room,
Byberry.
*City Archives of
Philadelphia.*

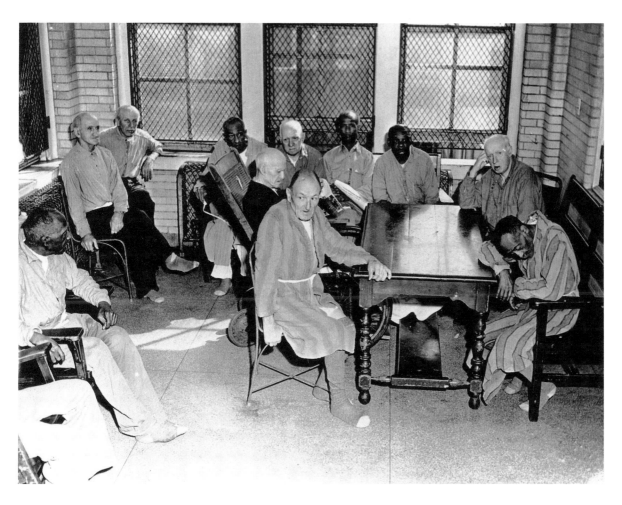

PHILADELPHIA GENERAL HOSPITAL, like many other large urban hospitals, maintained a facility for the diagnosis and evaluation of what were—in theory at least—recent acute psychiatric cases. Taken in 1945 for the *Philadelphia Evening Bulletin*, this image was labeled "Men Patients in Psychopathic Department." It suggests how little the care of the mentally disabled had changed. In their idleness, their unkempt appearance, and their general demeanor, these men resemble those who had passed through the wards of Blockley fifty years earlier.

84.

Psychopathic ward, Philadelphia General Hospital. *Temple University Urban Archives.*

THE EMERGENCE OF SCIENTIFIC MEDICINE:
THE PHYSICIAN'S NEW TOOLS

To THE MAJORITY of American men and women—and to many physicians—modern surgery seemed to represent the incarnation and triumph of scientific medicine. Antiseptic and later aseptic surgery allowed physicians to operate on parts of the body previously considered too dangerous to explore. Operations moved from the kitchen table and the private boarding house to the hospital operating theater, and the numbers of operations increased dramatically. At the Hospital of the University of Pennsylvania 209 operations were performed in 1880, by 1910 there were 2,067 surgical cases treated in the hospital, and by the 1940s the annual number reached almost 10,000.

Surgery played a pivotal role in bringing new patients to the hospital, helping transform it from a facility oriented toward the indigent chronically ill to one serving men and women from all social classes. Surgery also helped to make physicians the leading actors on this medical stage as hospital trustees increasingly ceded power and decision-making to medical professionals and trained administrators.

Earlier images of students observing in the surgical ampitheater illustrated the evolution of aseptic techniques and parallel advances in anesthesiology. Certainly much has changed since Dr. John Bower staged this sham operation scene at Blockley over a century ago. In this image the surgeons and nurses are without gowns and gloves, the room is not enclosed and is far from sterile, anesthesia consists of a hand-held ether cone, and the patient, head resting on a pillow, is held securely to the operating table by the physician's steady hand. Yet elements of the modern can be seen as well, from the overhead light source to the surgical instruments laid within easy grasp of the surgeon, who is shown saw in hand and seemingly ready to perform an amputation. The operating area is well staffed and generously stocked, with bowls, additional instruments, and drugs and bandages only a few steps away. However primitive this procedure appears in retrospect, it was operations such as this one, undertaken by skilled surgeons, that helped to transform the hospital into a modern institution, associated by both patients and physicians with the advanced technology that has come to seem indistinguishable from its fundamental identity.

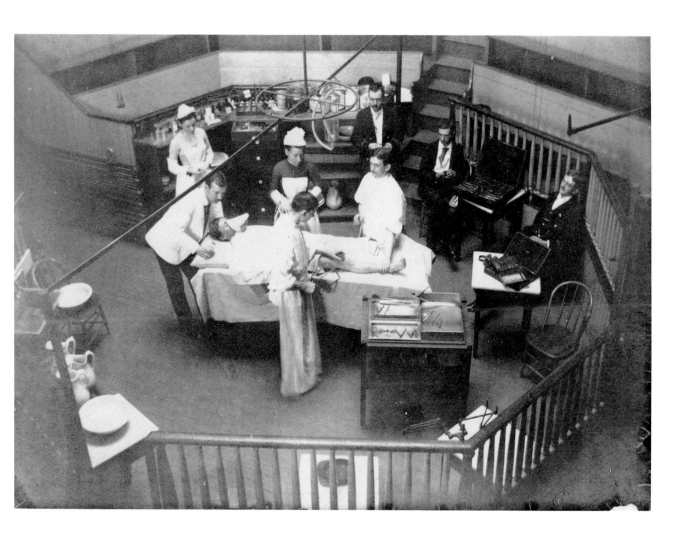

85.

Sham operation, Phila-
delphia General Hospital.
Historical Collections,
College of Physicians of
Philadelphia.

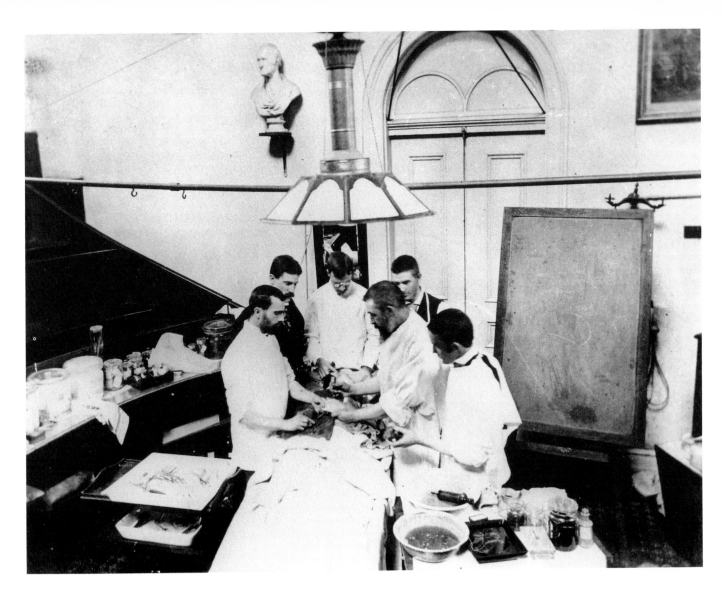

86.

Operation, Pennsylvania
Hospital.
*Pennsylvania Hospital
Archives.*

A BLOODIER, MORE realistic image, taken in 1894
at the Pennsylvania Hospital, shows the surgeons
with neither masks nor gloves, busy at work.

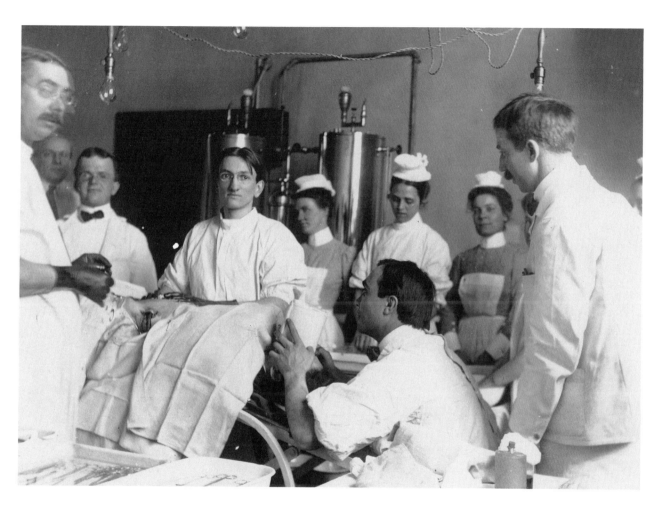

As the hospital became a place in which the body was invaded by an ever-proliferating array of diagnostic and therapeutic procedures, the photographic view shifted from the wide-angle image of the ampitheater to the close-up of the surgeon at work. Taken only a decade or so after the "sham operation" this image shows a surgical team at work in the Blockley operating room.

87.

Close-up of operation, Philadelphia General Hospital.
Center for the Study of the History of Nursing, School of Nursing, University of Pennsylvania.

88.

X-ray laboratory, Philadelphia Polyclinic. *University of Pennsylvania Archives.*

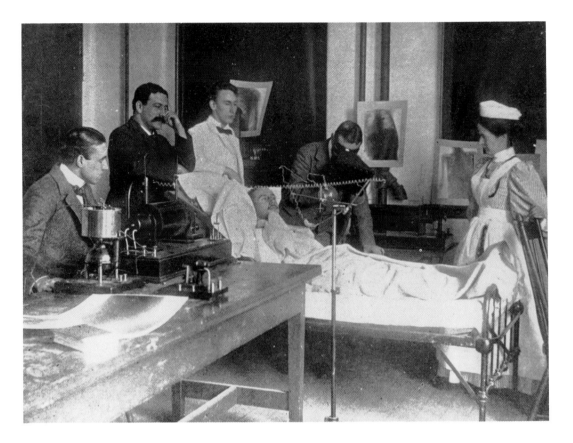

THE X-RAY ALLOWED visual access into the body: physicians could now see broken bones, for example, or skeletal abnormalities. Radiological apparatus became a critical part of the hospital's technical rationale, a reason why patients with fractures, kidney stones, imbedded foreign bodies, and congenital bone problems would need to visit the hospital for diagnosis and treatment. Incorporation of the new technology into medical practice took time, however. The Pennsylvania Hospital purchased a machine in 1897; ten years later it was still being employed only sporadically, as much out of curiosity as for practical diag-

nostic purposes. But eventually x-rays moved from the periphery to the center of hospital care, helping to change the way medicine was studied and practiced, the way patient records were kept, and even the way revenue flowed within the institution. Soon therapeutic as well as diagnostic uses were suggested for this new technology.

After a brief experimental period in which a variety of individuals, from photographers to physicians, operated pioneer x-ray units, most hospitals assigned responsibility to house officers. But as the images the machines produced became more critical to the practice of medicine, they

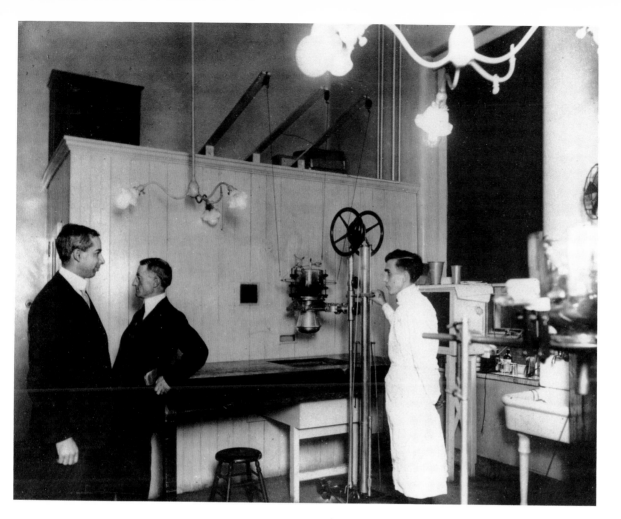

were read and often made by a new kind of specialist, the "roentgenologist." Just as novel technologies helped develop what we call "modern medicine," they also created hospital-based medical specialties and allied health professions.

This early photograph of the roentgen ray laboratory at the Philadelphia Polyclinic (now Graduate Hospital) displays both the machines and the images they created. Published in an annual report in 1896, only months after the first medical uses of the new rays, the photograph was clearly intended to show both to best advantage.

THIS 1913 PHOTOGRAPH shows the x-ray transformer and other radiology equipment at Hahnemann Hospital. To the right is pioneer technologist Arthur Morgan, who in 1921 founded the first school of x-ray technology in the United States. Morgan had been working as an orderly in the clinical laboratory and accident ward in 1911 when he was called for an interview with Dr. J. W. Frank, the head of the department of roentgenology and electric therapy. Recalling the meeting years later, Morgan said he had been asked to write his name, after which Frank looked up and said, "Alright, the job is yours."

89.

X-ray equipment, Hahnemann Hospital. *Archives, Hahnemann University.*

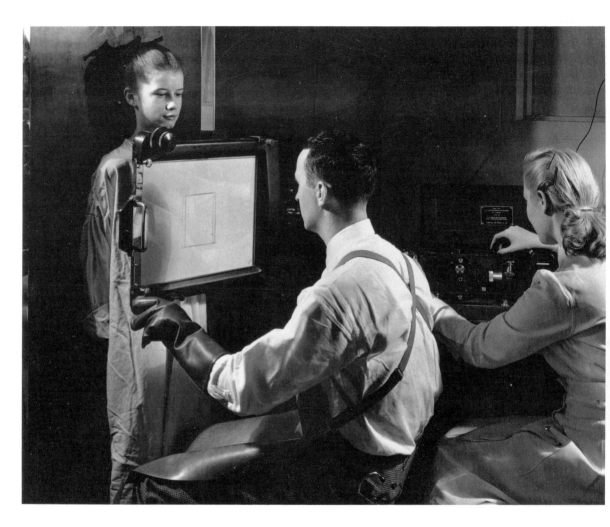

90.

X-ray laboratory, Hospital
of the Univeristy of
Pennsylvania.
University of Pennsyl-
vania Archives.

A 1938 PHOTOGRAPH from the x-ray laboratory at
the Hospital of the University of Pennsylvania
shows two diagnostic tools in use. The patient
stands behind a fluoroscope while the woman on
the right is operating an EKG unit.

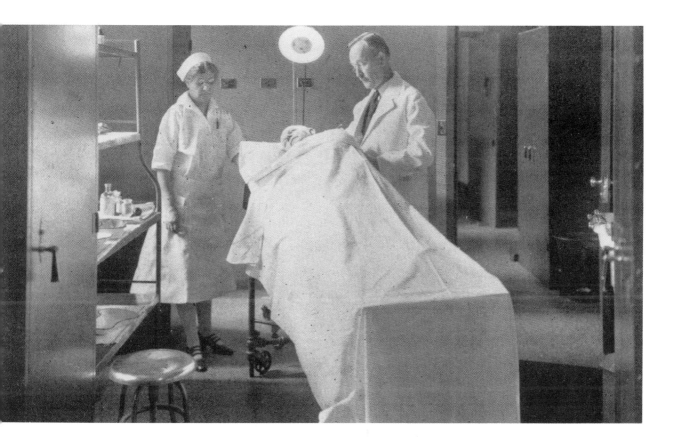

TREATING CANCER WAS perhaps the most widely utilized application of radiation therapy in early-twentieth-century medicine. Hahnemann Hospital was quick to establish a separate department of radium therapy, shown here in 1932.

91.

Radium therapy, Hahnemann Hospital. *Archives, Hahnemann University.*

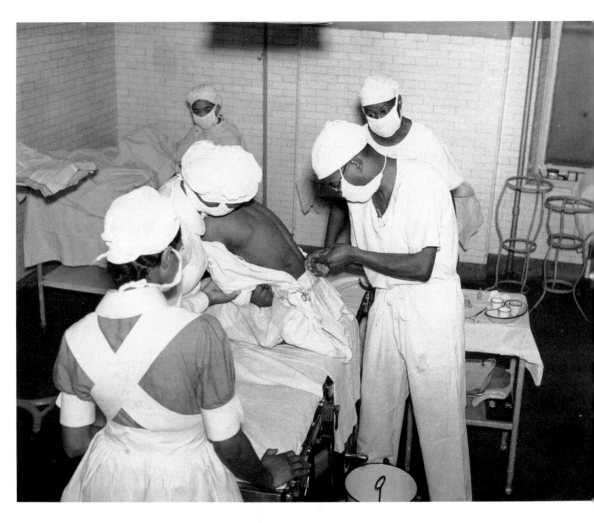

92.

Spinal tap.
Charles L. Blockson Afro-American Collection, Temple University.

THE SPINAL TAP, shown here, was a more invasive diagnostic procedure, which combined clinical and laboratory skills. Physicians examined the spinal fluid for color and clarity, chemically tested it for proteins, examined it under a microscope for red and white cells, and cultured it for bacteria. Among the diseases diagnosed with this test were meningitis, polio, and tertiary syphilis.

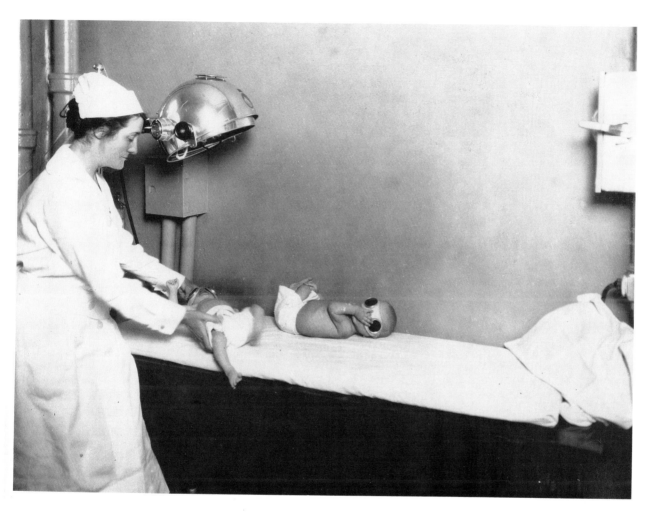

TREATMENT WITH ULTRA-VIOLET light, illustrated in this 1924 image from the Children's Hospital of Philadelphia, was once a means of treating rickets and was also used in managing dermatological ills.

93.

Light therapy, Children's Hospital of Philadelphia. *Children's Hospital of Philadelphia.*

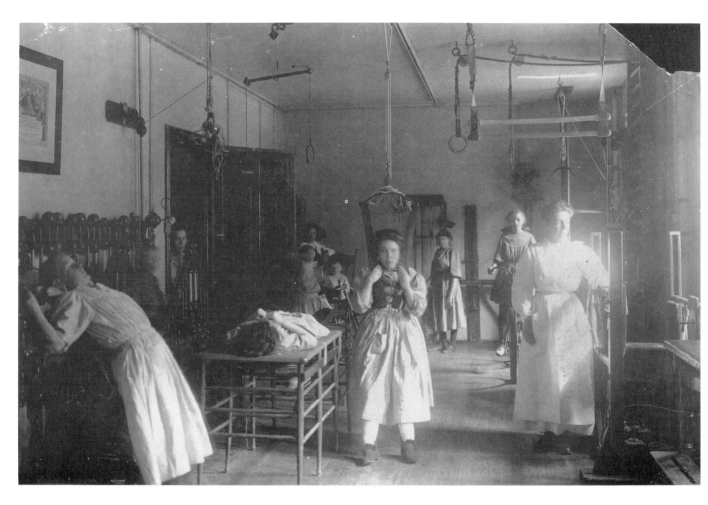

94.

Physical therapy, Hospital of the University of Pennsylvania.
University of Pennsylvania Archives.

THE VALUE OF physical therapy was widely recognized after World War I, and the advent of new physical therapy apparatus, operated by physicians and other trained personnel, soon made this an important part of medical care. A 1911 image from the Hospital of the University of Pennsylvania displays the gymnasium located in the orthopedic children's ward. The young women using the equipment seem more like students at a girls' school than hospital patients.

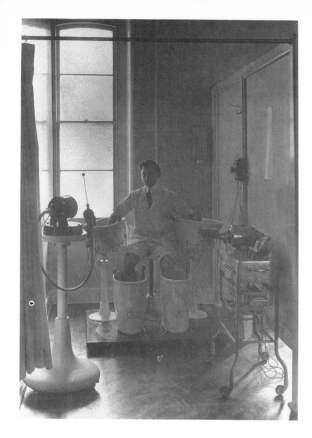

95.

Four-cell bath, Hospital of the University of Pennsylvania.
University of Pennsylvania Archives.

96.

Electric light cabinets, Hospital of the University of Pennsylvania.
University of Pennsylvania Archives.

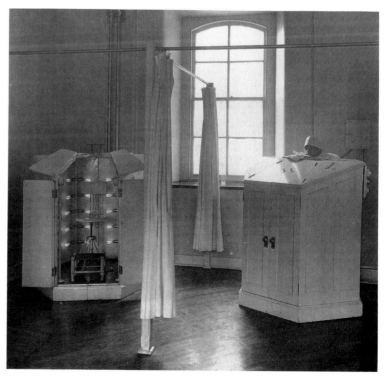

A MORE ELABORATE technology is demonstrated in these 1913 photographs from the hospital's physical therapy department. The first shows a four-cell bath, pantostat, and electric vibrator. The second shows two electric light cabinets, possibly used for the treatment of skin diseases.

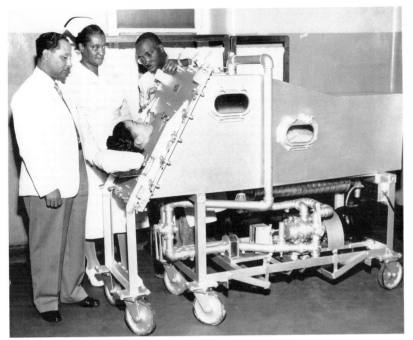

THESE IMAGES OF respirators, or "iron lungs," remind us of the polio epidemics in decades past and of the dependence of literally thousands of patients on these mechanical breathing devices. They also illustrate how the technology changed and improved over time. The first device pictured is a Drinker respirator from the 1930s; in the second photograph, dated 1942, donated respirators are being assembled at the Episcopal Hospital to be used there and in other area facilities.

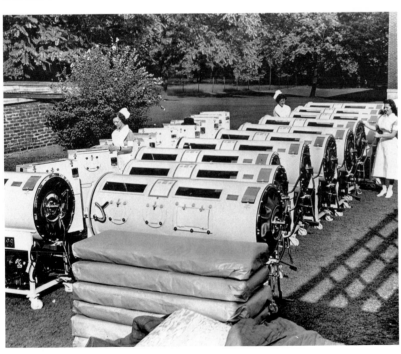

97.

Iron lung with patient.
Afro-American Historical and Cultural Museum.

98.

Iron lungs on lawn, Episcopal Hospital.
Temple University Urban Archives.

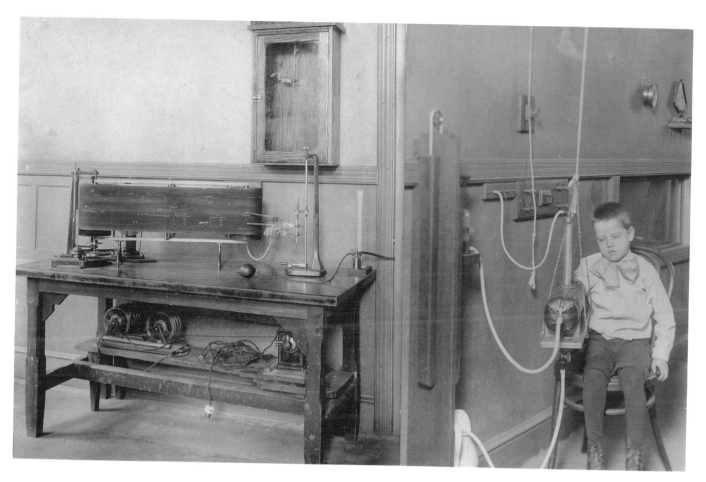

CLINICAL RESEARCH TRANSFORMED teaching hospitals as well as the medical school; laboratories were added and new biochemical, cytological, and physiological function tests developed as biomedical scientists sought to understand the mechanisms underlying clinical syndromes. After World War I, the previously shaky alliance between science and clinical medicine became more firmly established, and a career as "clinical investigator" became a viable option for an academically oriented minority among the medical elite. However, the inherent conflict between delivering care at the bedside and conducting investigative research in the laboratory has never been entirely resolved.

A 1904 photograph (actually two adjacent images) from the department of physiology at the Hospital of the University of Pennsylvania presents a laboratory experiment underway.

99.

Experiment with boy, Hospital of the University of Pennsylvania. *University of Pennsylvania Archives.*

100.

Experiment with stomach
thermometer, Hahnemann
University.
*Archives Hahnemann
University.*

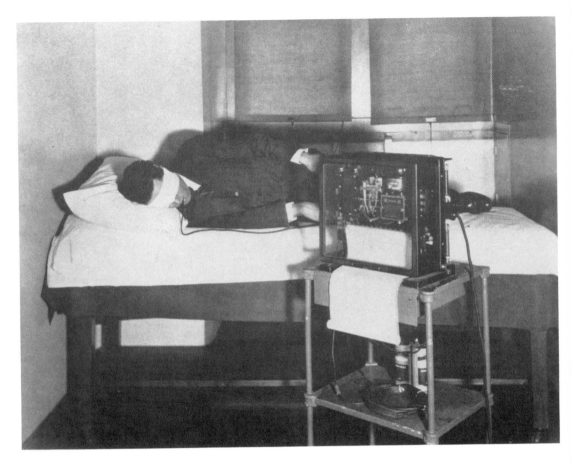

AN IMAGE FROM the Hahnemann Medical School
yearbook in 1932 shows a recording resistance
thermometer (designed for gastro-intestinal research), measuring the temperature of the stomach, upper intestine, and sigmoid as part of a
study of the influence on temperature of foods,
hot water bottles, ice bags, electric pads, and
other externally applied devices.

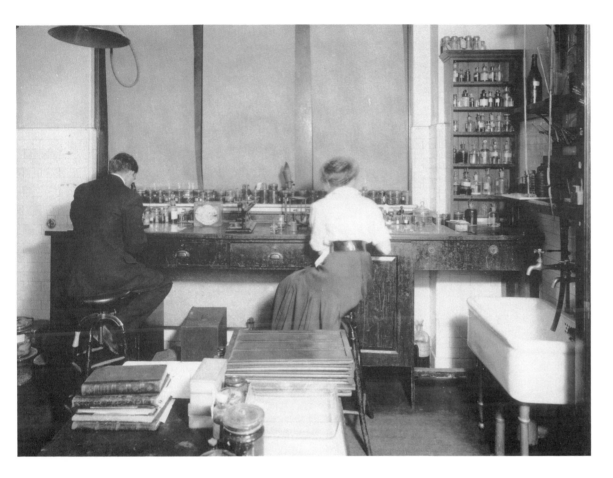

BY THE TWENTIETH century the chemical beaker
and the microscope were accepted tools of the
medical trade. Teaching hospitals became increasingly receptive to the work of biochemically
trained pathologists and clinical investigators.
Two images (here and on the next page) from the
Hospital of the University of Pennsylvania record
laboratories in a hospital setting. In facilities such
as these, physicians and a gradually increasing
number of basic scientists engaged in clinically
oriented research.

101.

Researchers, Hospital of
the University of Pennsylvania.
*University of Pennsyl-
vania Archives.*

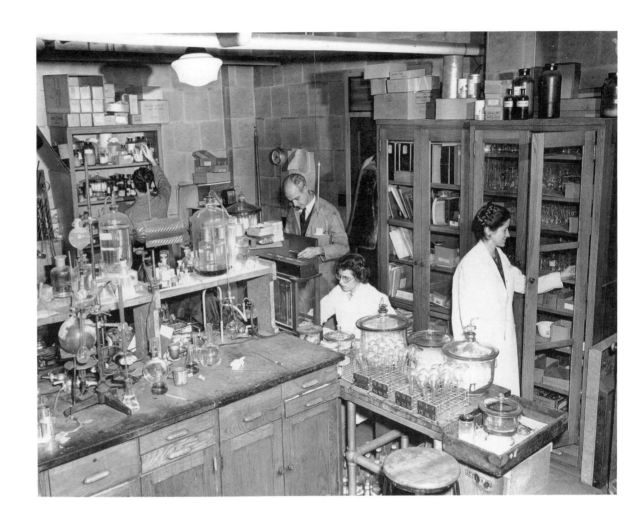

102.

Laboratory, Hospital of
the University of Penn-
sylvania.
*University of Pennsyl-
vania Archives.*

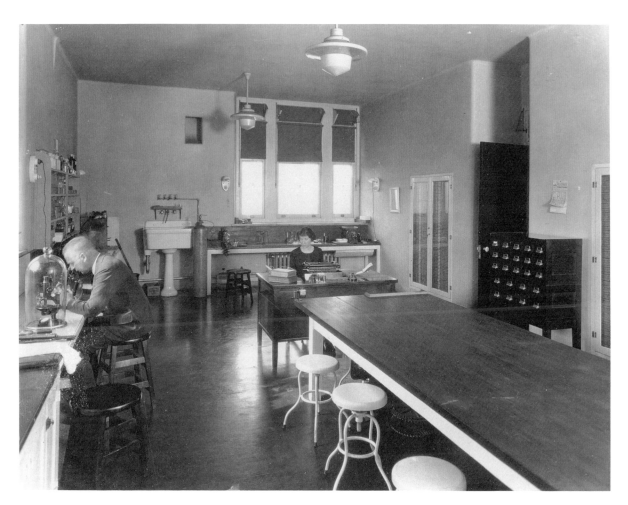

THE PICTURE OF the lone scientist at his microscope has long been a cultural cliché. Taken in
1924 at the Hospital of the University of Pennsylvania, this photograph exemplifies the place that
the laboratory came to hold in shaping the public
image of modern hospitals.

103.

Scientist at microscope,
Hospital of the University
of Pennsylvania.
*University of Pennsyl-
vania Archives.*

104.

Osler with body parts,
Philadelphia General
Hospital.
*Historical Collections,
College of Physicians of
Philadelphia.*

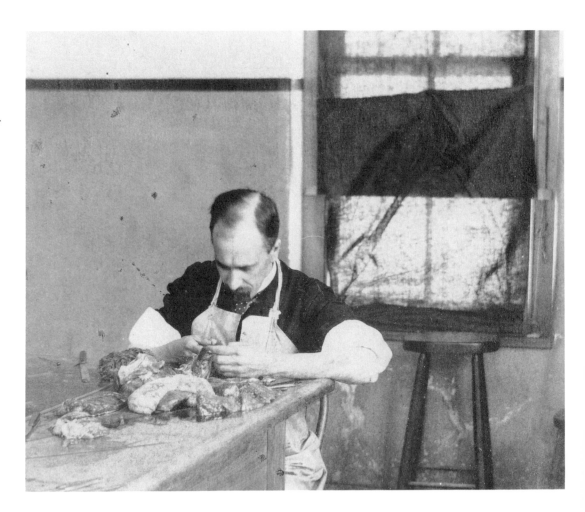

By the second quarter of the twentieth century pathology had become a broad field of inquiry encompassing chemical and experimental methods as well as studies of cell morphology and function.

In his biography of William Osler (1849–1919), Harvey Cushing describes his protagonist's "disinclination for a general practice" and his hours at Blockley, where "he would betake himself with a group of students to spend the afternoon making post-mortem examinations instead of sitting in his office awaiting patients." Photographed in the pathology laboratory at the Philadelphia General Hospital, where he regularly worked during his brief (1884–1888) but productive Philadelphia years, Osler symbolized the disciplined would-be clinical investigator.

In the second image, Osler (figure 11) bends over the cadaver. Among the other physicians

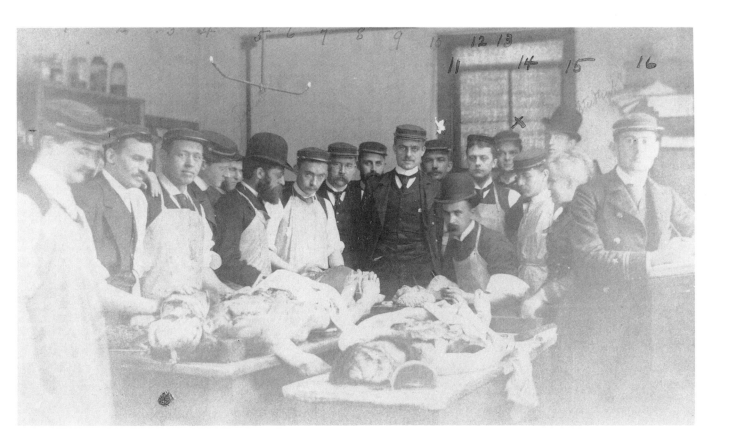

present are Charles Walter (1866–1891, figure 1),
William Beatty Jameson (1860–?, figure 3),
William T. Sharpless (1856–1947, figure 4),
Charles K. Mills (1845–1931, figure 5), Thomas
G. Ashton (1867–1933, figure 12), and August A.
Eshner (1862–1928, figure 15). The woman in the
figure is Amelia Weed Gilmore (1842–1928).

105.

Osler at autopsy, Phila-
delphia General Hospital.
*Center for the Study of
the History of Nursing,
School of Nursing, Uni-
versity of Pennsylvania.*

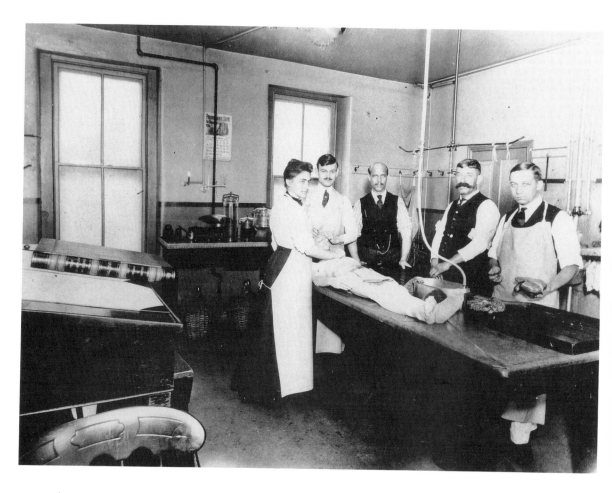

106.

Pathology laboratory,
Philadelphia General
Hospital.
*Historical Collections,
College of Physicians of
Philadelphia.*

ANOTHER PHOTOGRAPH OF a pathology laboratory
shows five physicians at the Philadelphia General
Hospital in 1903, as they remove organs from a
cadaver for study. The physicians are (from left
to right) Georgiana Walter, John Dyer, George
Taggart (?1867–1945), John Robinson, and
J. D. Blackwood (1881–1942).

AMBULANCE SERVICE

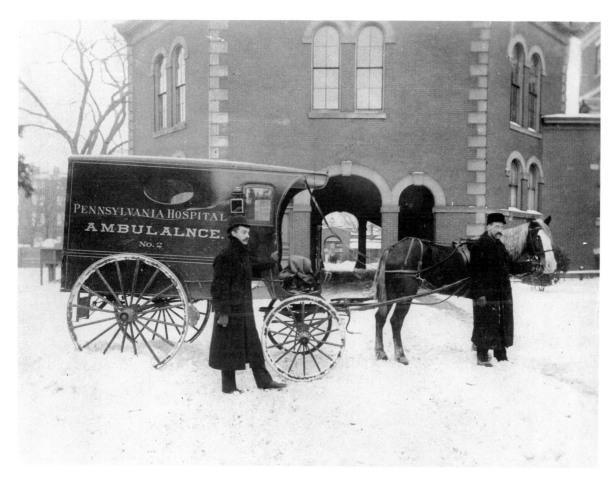

DURING THE CIVIL WAR, horse-drawn ambulances carried the sick and wounded to aid stations and hospitals. In the decades that followed their civilian counterparts responded to illnesses, accidents, and emergencies, transporting ambulance surgeons (fully equipped with medicine and instruments) to the patient and then carrying those needing further care to the hospital. With the hospital name emblazoned on their sides, ambulances also served as mobile advertisements.

Here Dick Howard, the ambulance driver from the Pennsylvania Hospital, poses alongside his horse. Howard came to the hospital for treatment of a broken arm and after his recovery stayed on as an employee for over fifty years. When the hospital purchased a motorized ambulance, he became a groundskeeper, Private hospitals assumed a paternalistic responsibility for their longtime employees.

107.

Dick Howard with horse-drawn ambulance, Pennsylvania Hospital. *Pennsylvania Hospital Archives.*

108.

Motorized ambulance,
Jefferson Hospital.
*Thomas Jefferson University, Scott Memorial
Library.*

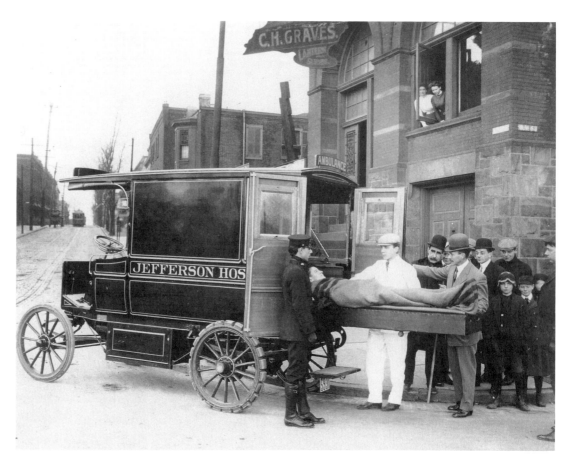

THE "MOTORIZED AMBULANCE" was only one of
the many non-medical technological developments that helped transform the twentieth-century
hospital. Among its advantages were the auto-
mobile's ability to stop quickly and to continue
operating in extremely hot weather. In this image,
the Thomas Jefferson University Hospital ambulance is loading a patient while a crowd gathers
to watch.

HOSPITALS PRODUCED HUNDREDS of pounds of
dirty laundry each day—soiled linens, gowns,
uniforms, and bandages. A growing understanding of the link between cleanliness and health
transformed the typical basement laundry from a
simple operation, such as the one pictured here at
Hahnemann Hospital at the turn of the century, to
the one below, from the Thomas Jefferson University Hospital.

Nineteenth-century hospital superintendents
and their administrative successors in the twentieth century laid down strict rules and rituals
for washing, bleaching, starching—designed to
prevent the transmission of disease to laundry
workers and patients and to ensure that the facility
operated at maximum efficiency. While these images suggest how hygienic standards and laundry
technology changed this hospital worksite, they
also show its enduring aspects.

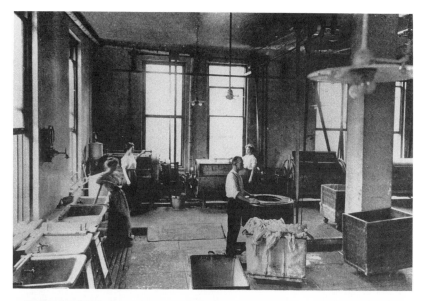

109.

Laundry, Hahnemann
Hospital.
*Archives, Hahnemann
University.*

110.

Laundry, Jefferson
Hospital.
*Thomas Jefferson Univer-
sity, Scott Memorial
Library.*

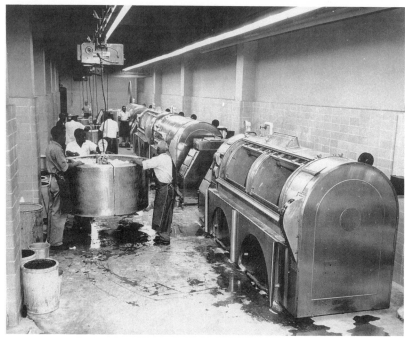

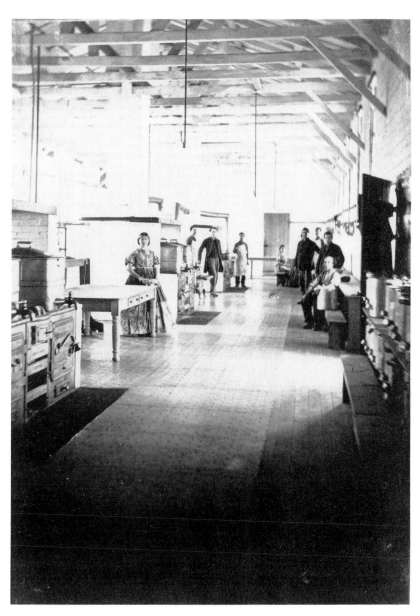

LIKE THE LAUNDRY, the hospital kitchen came to be operated according to self-consciously precise scientific and managerial principles. The "science of nutrition" determined what kind of meals patients would be served, while managerial standards imposed order and efficiency on the buying and apportioning of food.

In what is probably one of the earliest images of a hospital kitchen, this photograph shows the cooking department and staff of a Civil War hospital in 1862.

111.

Civil War hospital kitchen.
The Library Company of Philadelphia.

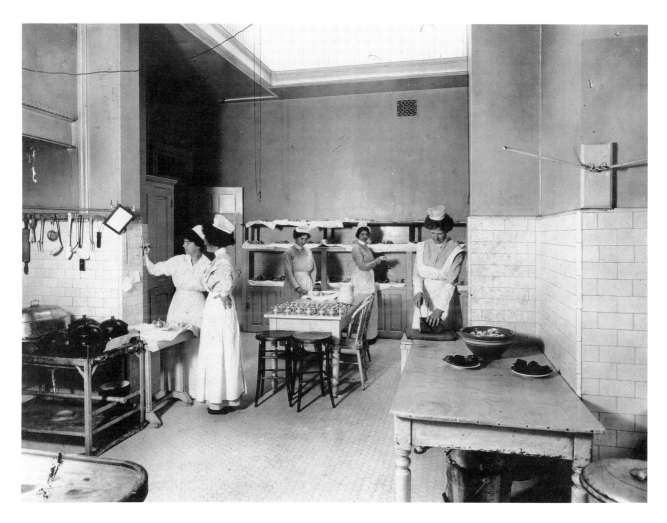

THIS IMAGE, FROM about 1910, shows nurses in
what is apparently a ward kitchen at the Hospital
of the University of Pennsylvania. As institutions
were rebuilt or modernized, central kitchens replaced such ward facilities and prepared meals for
the entire patient population.

112.

Ward kitchen, Hospital of
the University of Penn-
sylvania.
*University of Pennsyl-
vania Archives.*

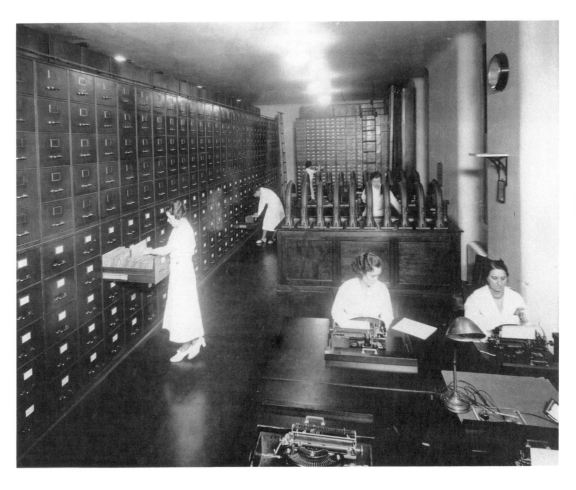

113.

Records room, Jefferson Hospital.
Thomas Jefferson University, Scott Memorial Library.

WHEN HOSPITALS SERVED as refuges for the sick poor, medical records were ordinarily maintained in ledgers that described in varying detail the personal life and medical complaints of each patient admitted. But with advances in medical diagnosis and treatment and with parallel efforts to impose a "scientific" and bureaucratic order on clincial data, the individual patients record replaced the register book. By the end of the nineteenth century physicians and nurses recorded information such as temperature and blood pressure on the medical record and appended, where relevant, the results of laboratory tests, x-ray readings, and other physical findings. Case records also listed drugs prescribed and procedures performed each day. The volume of data led to the creation of new types of hospital workers—medical secretaries and registrars—and to a new facility—the records room. Shown here is the Thomas Jefferson University Hospital records room after World War I.

PHARMACIES

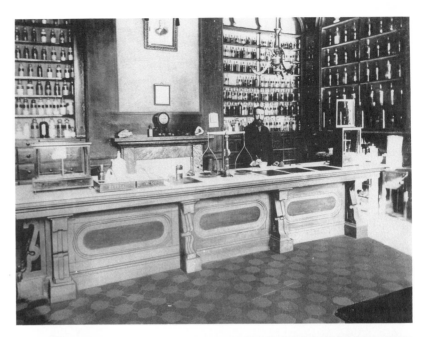

FROM THEIR EARLIEST beginnings, American hospitals had always housed pharmacies; in the late eighteenth and early nineteenth century the so-called pharmacist might be the only paid resident house officer. With increasing complexity and diversity of the materia medica, hospital pharmacies became larger and more recognizably modern. Their work load consisted largely of compounding and issuing prescriptions to an institution's numerous outpatients.

Pharmacies are instantly recognizable by their walls of medicine bottles. The first image shows the Pennsylvania Hospital pharmacy in the late nineteenth century. As the nation's first hospital the Pennsylvania Hospital also boasted having employed the nation's first hospital apothecary. The second image shows a busier and more modern pharmacy at the University of Pennsylvania.

114.

Pharmacy, Pennsylvania Hospital.
Pennsylvania Hospital Archives.

115.

Pharmacy, Hospital of the University of Pennsylvania.
University of Pennsylvania Archives.

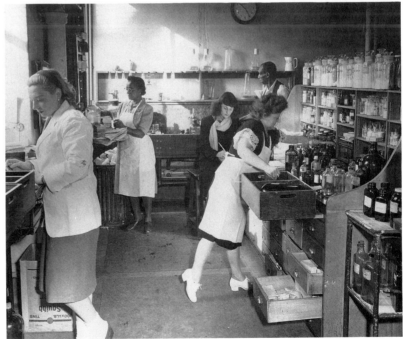

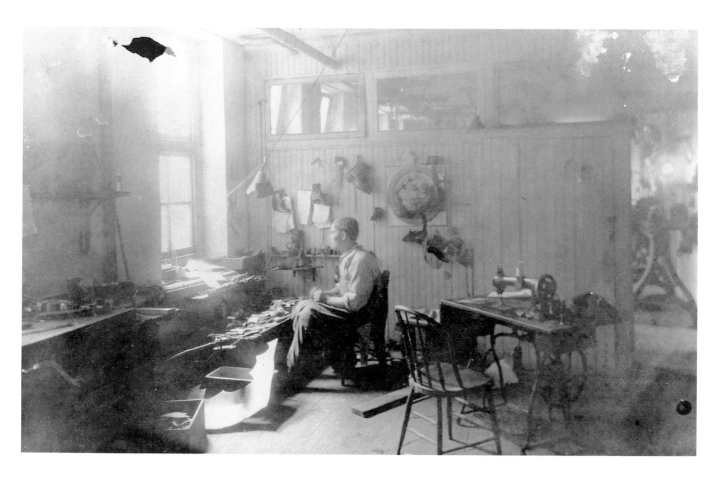

116.

Shoe shop, Hospital of
the University of Pennsylvania.
*University of Pennsyl-
vania Archives.*

WITH LARGE NUMBERS of patients admitted to
hospitals with chronic orthopedic complaints, it is
not surprising that some institutions maintained a
workshop on the premises to manufacture special
"appliances" as is depicted in this image of the
Hospital of the University of Pennsylvania shoe
shop, which opened in 1884. Most hospitals with
orthopedic services housed departments in which
braces and crutches were made and provided to
both in- and outpatients.

THREE

Health in the Community

PROTECTING THE HEALTH of Philadelphians in the half-century before World War II encompassed a wide range of public and voluntary activities, among them the collection of vital statistics, the building of sewers, the killing of pests, and the provision of care for pregnant women and their babies. Other efforts included isolating the carriers of communicable diseases, administering quarantines, inspecting food, maintaining a clean water supply, collecting and disposing of garbage, cleaning streets, offering industrial hygiene programs, and initiating health education campaigns. Although it is hard to quantify their demographic impact with precision, these endeavors almost certainly helped to lower morbidity and mortality rates and to improve the quality of life for all Philadelphians.

What spurred public health reform? Sometimes it took epidemics (both real and threatened) to stimulate action; in other cases individual reformers and organizations led the way. Beginning in the late nineteenth century, sanitarians, public officials, engineers, and health professionals all grappled with the compelling problems posed by an increasingly dense and seemingly pathogenic urban environment. As the population of Philadelphia grew, as new immigrants arrived, as sweatshops proliferated, and as industries expanded, earlier arrangements for coping with the city's health needs proved inadequate.

An embryonic public health program was in place by the end of the 1870s; and such efforts were sharpened and inspired by the periodic recrudescence of infectious diseases in the next two decades. Not all the city's problems were tackled successfully, but by World War I a municipal health regimen had been established; the city's public health programs would have been recognizable to a late-twentieth-century eye.

Photographers were deeply engaged in many aspects of the public health endeavor. Some documented the filthy conditions in which many Philadelphians lived, worked, and fell ill. Others created images used in educational campaigns designed to change individual behavior. Less frequently, photographers recorded public activities, such as the laying of sewer pipes or the hauling of trash.

Photographs capture three vital components of the increasingly self-conscious public health enterprise. First, they chronicled the impact of the germ theory and of bacteriology on municipal policy. We see milk being pasteurized, children being inoculated, families being quarantined, and workers having chest x-rays taken. At the same time, late-nineteenth- and early-twentieth-century photographs show how older notions of sanitation and hygiene persisted, reflecting a widely assumed "filth theory" of disease and a parallel, and not entirely unrelated, commitment to an aesthetic of civic "decency." Streets were swept, ashes hauled away, and vacant lots cleared of rubbish.

Second, the photographs display the influence of politics on medicine— as exemplified by the pictures of squalid slums and sickly children disseminated by reformers or the images of well-publicized clean-up parades. This theme is reinforced in the disproportionately large number of pictures of infants and children. Politicians, reformers, and health professionals alike agreed that saving the young offered a genuine opportunity to improve society. Work with children promised results, even if their degraded parents seemed alien and little amenable to moral or physical reform.

A third, less pronounced theme is the heterogeneity of the public health work force. It included a good many Philadelphians who were neither doctors nor nurses. Employees of the city's public works, health, welfare, and water departments were the foot soldiers in Philadelphia's campaign to protect the public's health. While their stories are often omitted from written accounts, their labors are visible in many of these photographs.

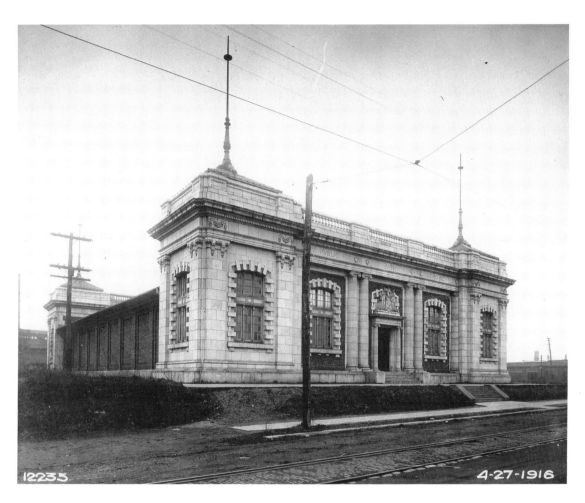

IN THE SECOND annual report (1878) of the Pennsylvania Free Dispensary for Skin Diseases, Dr. John V. Shoemaker (1852–1910) called for the city to establish free baths "to mitigate the suffering of the poor and lessen disease." Many of those arriving at the dispensary, he lamented, had "never bathed their entire body or had gone for years without doing so." In response to such conditions, Philadelphia, like other cities, built and maintained public baths, among them the Tacony municipal bath house, shown here.

117.

Tacony bath house.
City Archives of Philadelphia.

118.

Shvitz bath.
*City Archives of
Philadelphia.*

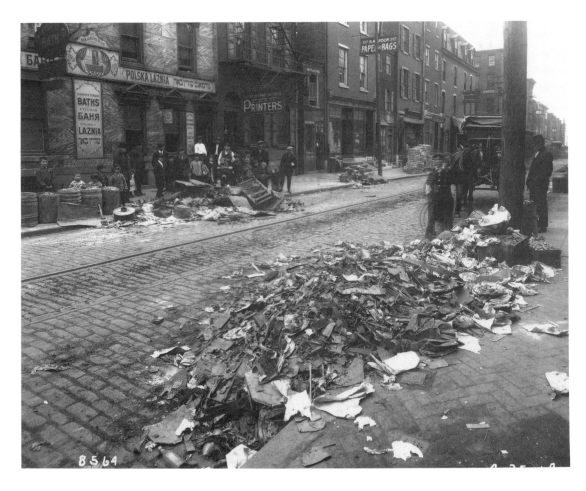

SOME CITIZENS PREFERRED, for religious or cultural reasons, to frequent private bath houses. This one, apparently a traditional Jewish "shvitz" (sweat or steam) bath operated by Sol Goodman, was located on Vine Street and catered to an Eastern European clientele. A sign in English proclaims it a "Russian & Turkish" bath, a sign in Russian labels it a "Russian Bath" a Polish sign calls it a Polish Bath, and the sign in Yiddish reads "Shvitz Bath." Other signs, in Yiddish and English, designate the entrance for men. For immigrants living in tenements with a water pump on the ground floor or in cold water flats, a visit to the bath house was necessary for maintaining personal cleanliness. It was also a social occasion.

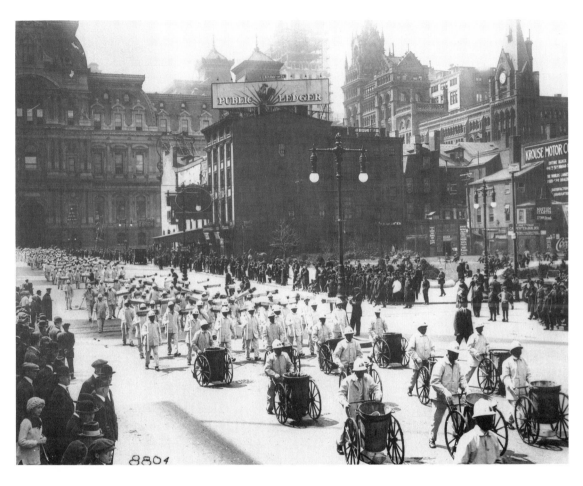

THE CITY WAS aware of its sanitation problems
and rallied both citizens and workers to duty with
a "clean-up week" in 1914. As a prelude to this
civic event, over two thousand city street cleaners
with their horse-drawn equipment paraded up
Broad Street before the mayor and other city officials. Those carrying large brooms were dubbed
"white wings." In the 1920s the city hired private
contractors to clean the city's 1,600 miles of paved
streets.

119.

Clean-up parade.
*City Archives of
Philadelphia.*

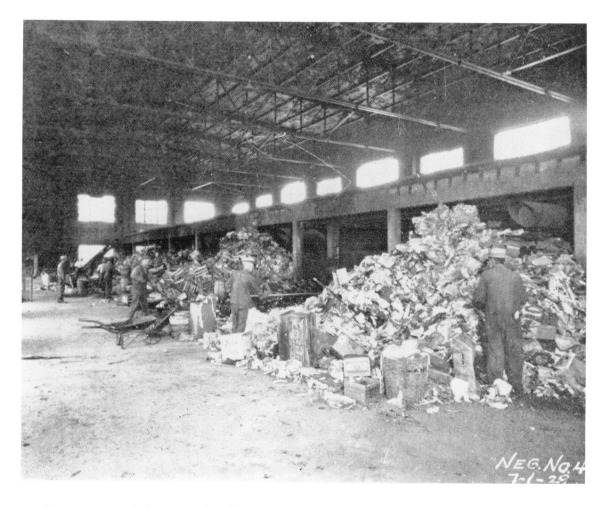

120.

Sorting floor of city incinerator.
Historical Collections, College of Physicians of Philadelphia.

IN ADDITION TO the brooms and trash cans the city employed fleets of horses and later "motor-driven" ash collectors and trash trucks. Garbage and trash were carted away for sorting and disposal. This image portrays the sorting floor at one of the city's incinerators.

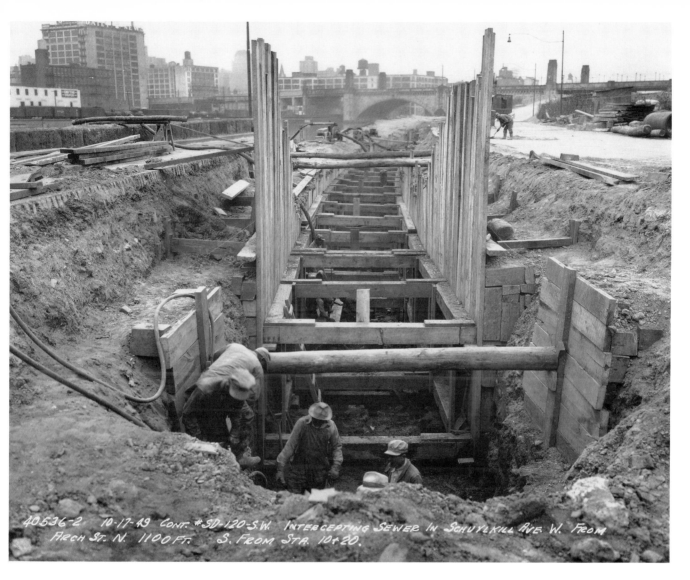

40536-2   10-17-49 Cont. #SD-120-S.W.   Intercepting Sewer in Schuylkill Ave. W. From
Arch St. N. 1100 FT.   S. From STA. 10+20.

SEWAGE DISPOSAL WAS another municipal responsibility. Under construction in this image is the intercepting sewer in Schuylkill Avenue. Civic pride and a new sense of minimal civic propriety allied themselves with a fear of typhoid and other water-borne diseases to encourage sewer construction. In 1906, when typhoid cases peaked in Philadelphia and filtration of the water supply had not yet been completed, there were 9,721 cases of the disease and 1,063 deaths. By the 1930s, when filtration had been completed and typhoid carriers systematically placed under the supervision of the Board of Health, annual deaths typically numbered fewer than twenty.

121.

Sewer construction.
City Archives of Philadelphia.

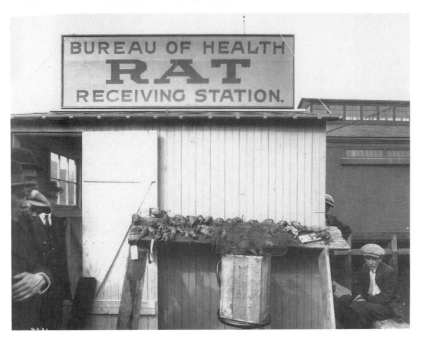

PEST CONTROL CONSTITUTED yet another important aspect of the city's multifaceted campaign to prevent or eradicate disease. Rats had been feared urban dwellers even before the discovery that their fleas spread bubonic plague. Philadelphia's efforts to solve the problem included a program that, as the poster indicates, offered a bounty of five cents each for live rats and two cents each for dead ones delivered to the rat receiving station on Delaware Avenue. In later years rat tunnels were gassed with carbon monoxide and escaping rats clubbed to death by city exterminators. Despite increasingly sophisticated efforts to annihilate them, rats remain one of the seemingly unavoidable features of city life.

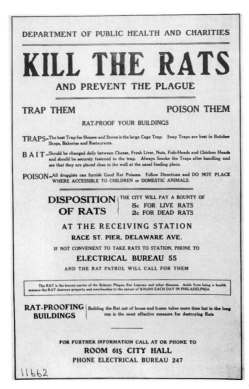

122.

Rat receiving station.
City Archives of Philadelphia.

123.

"Kill rats" poster.
City Archives of Philadelphia.

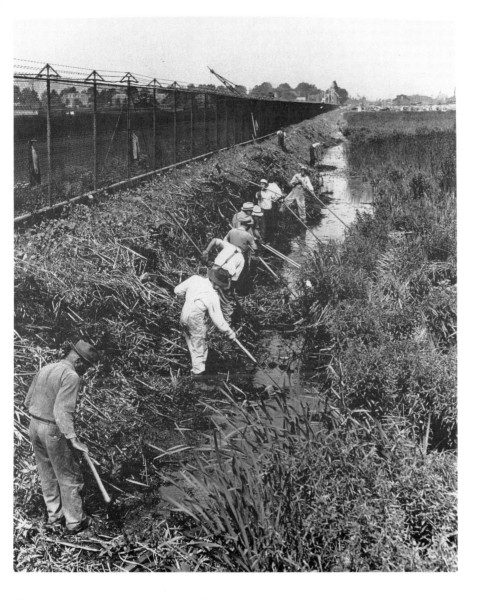

124.

Drainage channel.
Temple University Urban Archives.

CERTAIN MOSQUITOES ALSO carried disease; the insect's role in spreading malaria had been known since the end of the nineteenth century. In this image, employees of the city's public works department are deepening a drainage channel in an effort to control mosquitoes.

IN RESPONSE TO alarming infant mortality rates, late-nineteenth-century American public health advocates initiated a variety of preventive measures. At the municipal level they worked to supply clean water and to pass laws requiring the pasteurization of milk. Individuals with measles, mumps, scarlet fever, and other communicable diseases were quarantined in their homes. Immunization programs were begun in schools and special classrooms provided for those deemed "pre-tubercular." In slum neighborhoods reformers concentrated on "baby saving." This comprehensive program included prenatal care, instruction for mothers in feeding and rearing their babies, sick and well baby care at local clinics, home care by visiting nurses, and the provision of pasteurized milk.

125.

Baby Saving Station. *Center for the Study of the History of Nursing, School of Nursing, University of Pennsylvania.*

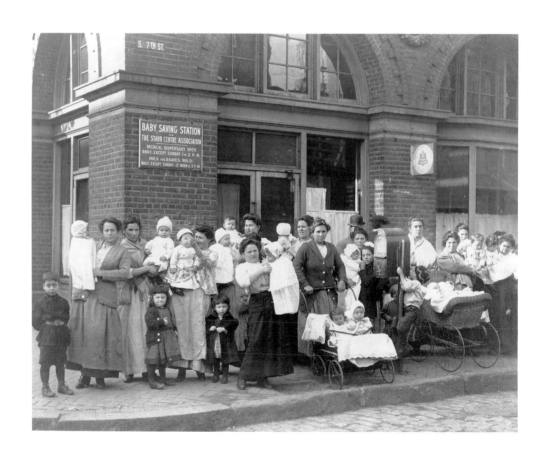

IN SOUTH PHILADELPHIA the Starr Centre Association, an organization dedicated to providing educational and medical as well as social services to the poor, sold pasteurized milk for one cent a bottle at its Baby Saving Station. As the sign indicates, families were also offered the services of physicians and visiting nurses, for the fees listed.

126.

Starr Centre poster. *Center for the Study of the History of Nursing, School of Nursing, University of Pennsylvania.*

⋆ STARR CENTRE
725-727-729 LOMBARD STREET

MILK for Babies for Sale Daily,
I cent per bottle,
12 to 5 P. M.

DISPENSARY Open Mondays,
Wednesdays *and* Fridays
2 P. M. to 3 P. M.

DOCTOR in charge, First advice as to milk—Free.
ADVICE TO PATIENTS 10c.
HOME CALLS   -   -   50c.
Special Rates—Rainy Day Society 25c.

NURSE will give care to sick for 10c.
PER VISIT IN THE HOMES.

Try the milk for sick or poorly nourished babies.
The milk is mixed with lime water, barley water, Etc.

DOES your Baby need our help? Remember condensed milk, tea or coffee, milk diluted with Schuylkill water, are bad for babies.

Last year we sold 361,807 bottles of milk to more than eleven hundred babies.

127.

Crippled children's
school.
*Center for the Study of
the History of Nursing,
School of Nursing, Uni-
versity of Pennsylvania.*

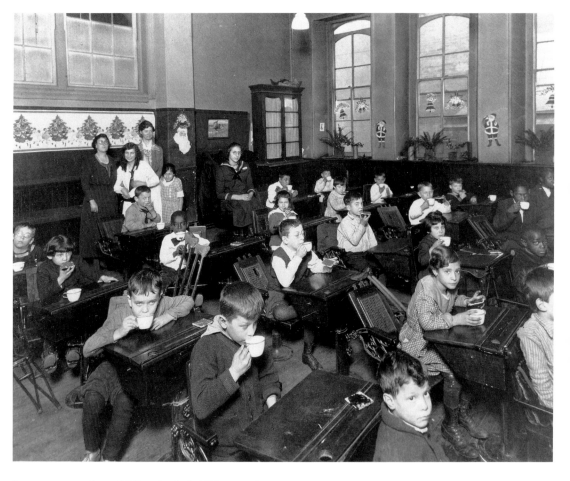

IN THIS IMAGE from 1917, crippled children at the
McCall Annex School are enjoying their penny
lunch.

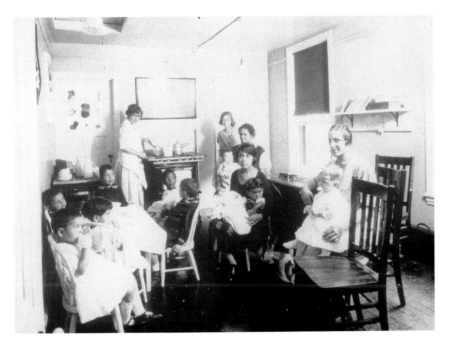

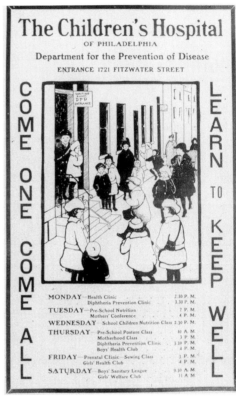

THE SOCIAL SERVICE division of the Children's Hospital of Philadelphia, the Department for the Prevention of Disease, offered clinics and classes for mothers and children as well as providing visiting nurses to the neighborhood. Much of its work was educational, including the organization of a girls' health club and a boys' sanitary league. The photograph appears to record one of the early childhood nutrition classes.

128.

Department for the Prevention of Disease, Children's Hospital. *Historical Collections, College of Physicians of Philadelphia.*

129.

Children's Hospital poster. *Historical Collections, College of Physicians of Philadelphia.*

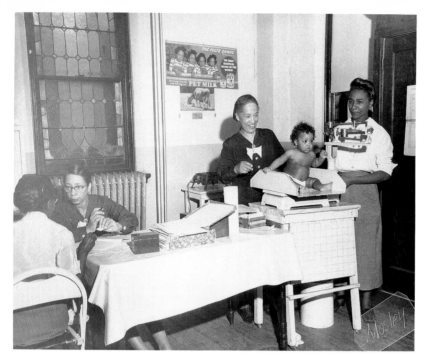

HEALTH PROGRAMS FOR children were provided at a number of sites, including hospitals, schools, settlement houses, and churches. The first image appears to be a well child program; the site is unidentified. The second image, probably taken at the Christian Street YMCA, shows a group of young men ready to undergo medical examinations.

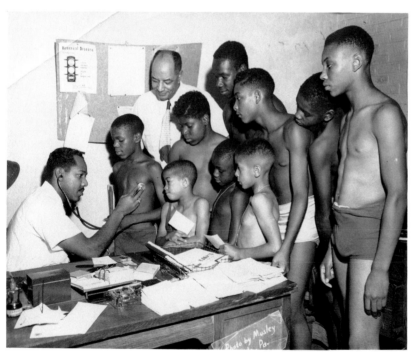

130.

Well child visit.
Charles L. Blockson Afro-American Collection, Temple University.

131.

YMCA examination.
Charles L. Blockson Afro-American Collection, Temple University.

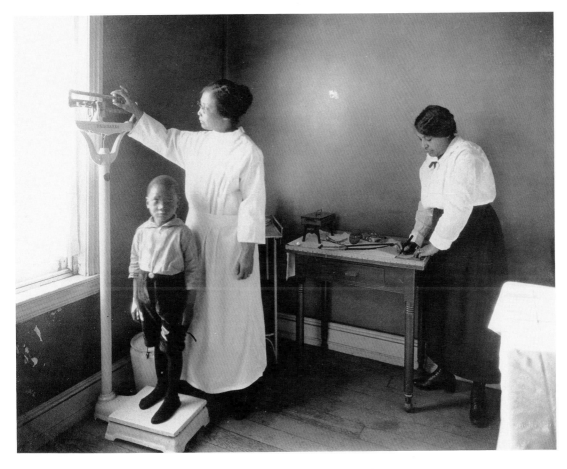

132.

Check-up at day nursery.
*Temple University Urban
Archives.*

PRE-SCHOOL CHILDREN attending some of the organized day nurseries throughout the city received
regular medical attention and health education.
This photograph, possibly from the Benezet Day
Nursery, depicts a young girl undergoing her
weekly check-up.

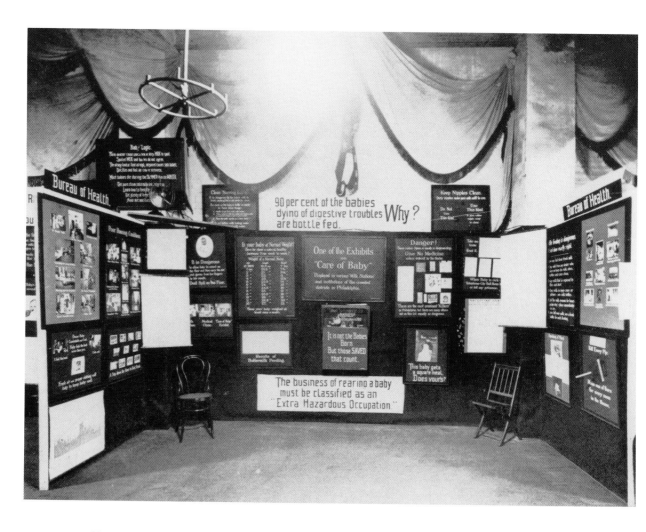

133.

Philadelphia Milk Show.
*Historical Collections,
College of Physicians of
Philadelphia.*

HEALTH EDUCATION PROGRAMS ranged from one-to-one efforts by public health nurses to instruct mothers in infant care to city-wide exhibitions. Among the latter was the 1911 Philadelphia Milk Show, which offered exhibits, lectures, and contests designed to stimulate a demand for high-quality milk. Over 110,000 Philadelphians at-tended the eight-day show. Its motto, "To Enlighten—Not to Frighten," suggests the public health workers' strategy; a variety of exhibits underlined the deadly effects of unclean or adulterated milk, while others featured health measures that could assure its quality.

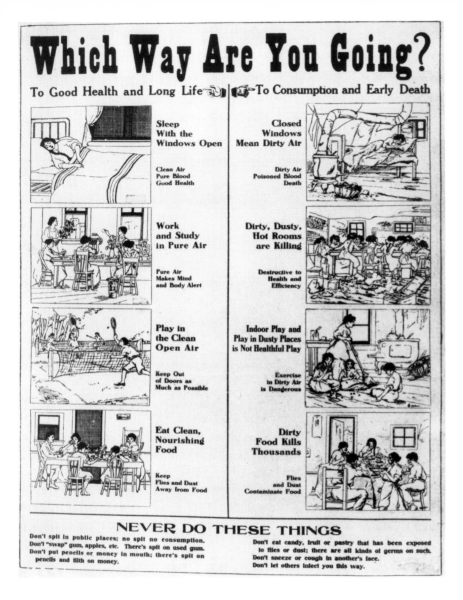

134.

Consumption poster.
*City Archives of
Philadelphia.*

This public health poster also offers the keys to
good health and a long life. A close look at the
illustrations reveals that the road to consumption
and early death was paved not just with dirty food
and air, dusty rooms, and indoor play, but with
poverty.

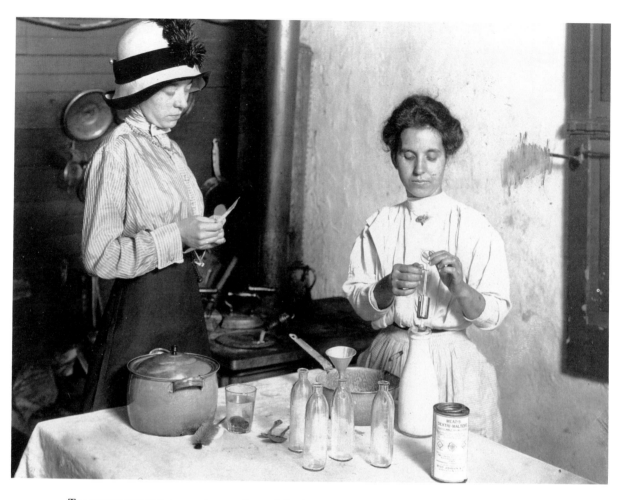

135.

Visiting nurse with mother.
Center for the Study of the History of Nursing, School of Nursing, University of Pennsylvania.

TEACHING MOTHERS HOW to care for and feed their babies properly was one of the major activities undertaken by visiting nurses. Here a nurse from the Starr Centre was photographed teaching a mother how to prepare her baby's milk.

REFORMERS, UNION LEADERS, and medical professionals were also concerned with work-related illness and death. They advocated factory inspection laws, controls on exposure to fumes, dust, and dangerous chemicals, and rules limiting the number of hours women and children could be employed. In some industries, railroads most prominently, it was standard practice in the late nineteenth century to maintain an industrial hospital or to endow a bed or beds in the local community hospital. In other instances, employee dispensaries grew into full-scale hospitals. John B. Stetson, the hat manufacturer, for example, opened a small dispensary for the benefit of Stetson company employees in the nearby North Fourth Street Union Mission. Eventually the dispensary started serving employees' family members and then neighborhood families, and finally evolved into the Union Mission Hospital, which after moving into new accommodations in 1905 became the Stetson Hospital.

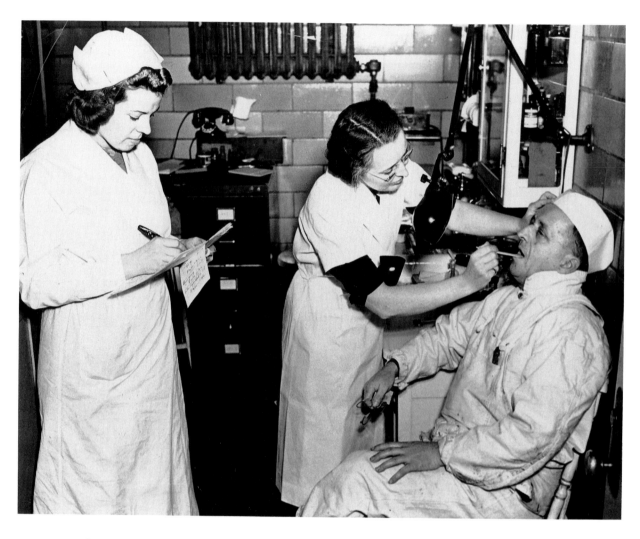

136.

Examination at packing plant.
Temple University Urban Archives.

IN THE TWENTIETH century a number of industries opened dispensaries or infirmaries at the work site. Pictured in a 1940 photograph is the dispensary maintained at a Philadelphia packing plant and staffed by a visiting nurse from the United Charities' Agency.

WARTIME MOBILIZATIONS HELPED to bring the issues of industrial hygiene into broader public view. The American worker was now a functional part of the military, and safety on the job was linked to homefront production needs as never before. In a time of labor shortage and high output needs, injuries cost money.

Industrial medicine had a well-established tradition in the nineteenth century; few photographs of these early activities are available. But when the nation went to war photographers were there to take pictures that would link industrial hygiene to public morale. Although many of the images can be labeled "propaganda," they are nevertheless revealing, documenting both industrial hygiene and, in some cases, the ways in which women began taking over jobs once held exclusively by men.

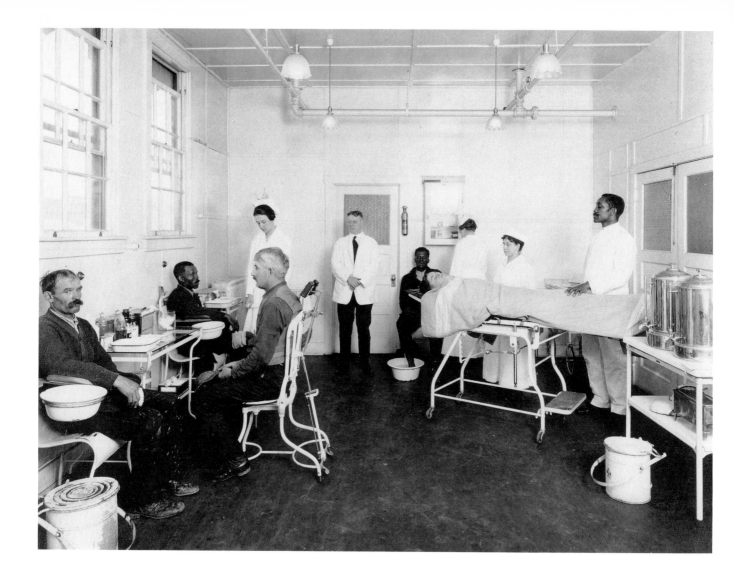

137.

First aid room, shipyard.
Atwater Kent Museum.

SHORTLY AFTER THE beginning of World War I, the American International Shipbuilding Corporation constructed the nation's largest shipyard at Hog Island. For a few short years the shipyard launched vessels at a record-breaking pace, employing as many as 26,000 workers each day. To meet the health needs of its labor force the company built a small surgical hospital and maintained the first aid facility shown here.

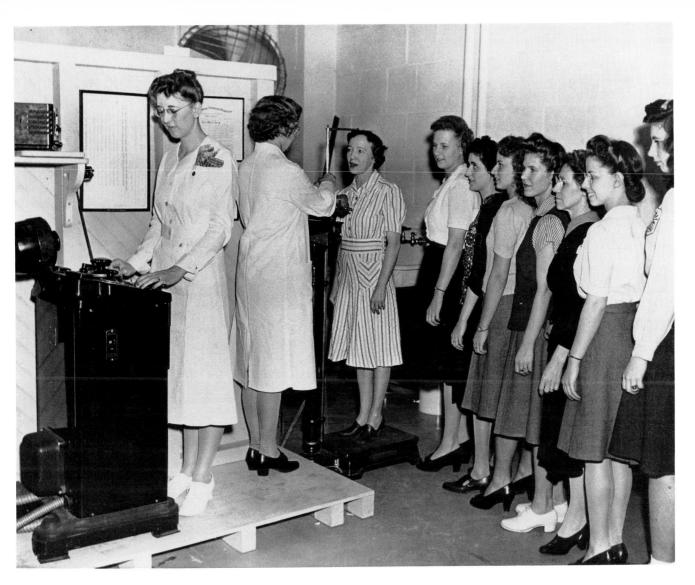

WORLD WAR II also led to intensified public health campaigns. Industrial hygiene efforts expanded tremendously; for example, the number of public health nurses employed in industry doubled, and widespread efforts to disseminate health information on the job and to detect and prevent disease were soon underway. Here civilian workers from the Frankford Arsenal line up for their free chest x-ray examinations, sponsored jointly by the local anti-tuberculosis association and the tuberculosis division of the Department of Public Health.

138.

Chest x-rays, Frankford Arsenal.
Temple University Urban Archives.

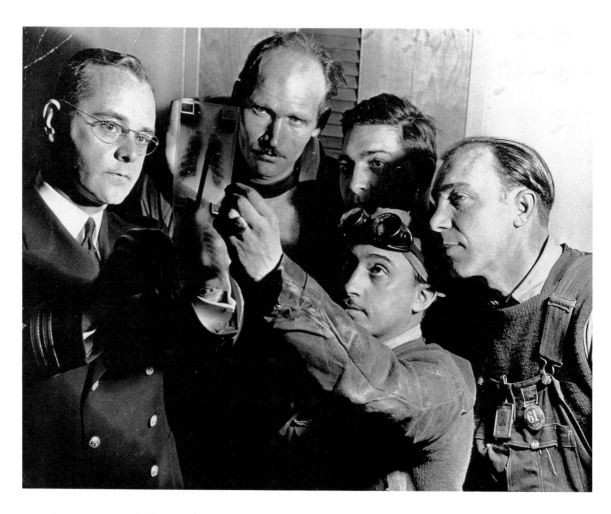

139.

Men holding up x-ray picture, Philadelphia Navy Yard.
Temple University Urban Archives.

IN THIS IMAGE civilian employees at the Philadelphia Navy Yard are shown after a visit to the "U.S.S. X-Ray." Chest x-rays were used primarily to screen for tuberculosis.

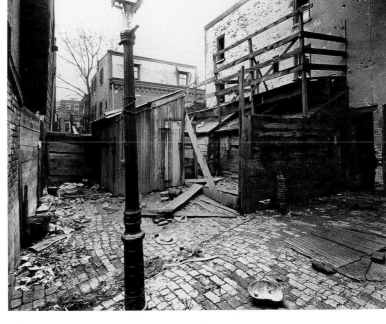

REFORMERS AND PHOTOGRAPHERS recorded a variety of the city's sanitation and hygiene problems on their visits to poor neighborhoods. The president of the Philadelphia Housing Commission noted in 1913 that the city had "200,000 people housed in alley dwellings, amid insanitation, on unsewered streets, with foul privy vaults abounding, or in over-crowded and poorly ventilated rooms, in converted tenements or rear dwellings, deprived of adequate light, or eating, cooking and sleeping in cellars and attics."

The Octavia Hill Association, a housing reform group, took before-and-after pictures of the housing it restored. Here is a dwelling in 1904 before being cleaned, and after. The third image of an alley dwelling (see next page) was created for the Philadelphia Housing Association.

140.

Franklin Court before purchase by Octavia Hill Association.
Temple University Urban Archives.

141.

Franklin Court after purchase and repair.
Temple University Urban Archives.

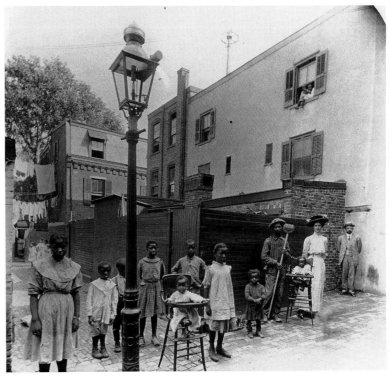

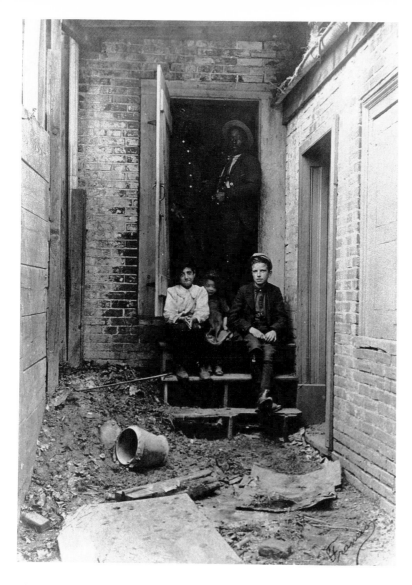

PHILADELPHIA'S DEPARTMENT OF Public Health and Charities also took an interest in housing issues relating to public health. The first photograph is from a tenement inspection. Residents not yet hooked up to the sewer line were required to follow the regulations issued by the Board of Health regarding the maintenance of privies.

142.

Alley dwelling.
Temple University Urban Archives.

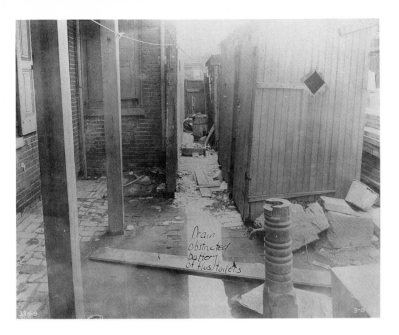

Drain
Obstructed
Battery
of Flus toilets

143.

Privies.
*Temple University Urban
Archives.*

144.

Privy rules.
*City Archives of
Philadelphia.*

Department of Public Health and Charities

RULES GOVERNING THE SANITARY MAINTENANCE
OF PRIVY VAULTS AND PRIVY HOUSES
IN THE CITY OF PHILADELPHIA

1. The occupants of premises will be held responsible for the maintenance of privy houses or closets in a sanitary condition and free from damage, except such as result from ordinary use.

2. Privy houses or closets shall be maintained in a clean and sanitary condition.

3. All openings in seats shall be provided with covers. A block shall be so arranged that the seat covers will fall into place when seat is not in use.

4. Wash water, garbage, kitchen slops, etc., shall not be emptied into privy wells.

5. The discharges from any person suffering from typhoid fever, dysentery, or other serious bowel disease, shall not be deposited in any privy well without being previously disinfected in the manner prescribed by the Bureau of Health.

6. Privy wells shall be cleaned, when their contents come to within three (3) feet of the ground level, and at other times when deemed necessary by the Bureau of Health, and shall be frequently treated with lime to prevent their becoming foul.

7. When a privy well is in need of cleaning, it shall be immediately reported by the tenant to the owner or agent and to the Bureau of Health.

8. Doors of privy houses and closets shall not be left open. They shall be so arranged that they will return into the closed position.

9. Doors shall be securely attached by hinges of such size as to properly support the weight of the door at all times.

10. All other openings in the privy houses or closets, except the doors, shall be tightly screened with screens not less than fourteen (14) meshes to the inch.

11. A supply of unslacked lime shall be kept on hand in each privy house or closet and shall be frequently applied to the contents of the privy well.

12. The privy house or closet shall be kept in good repair, and if any part shall become decayed or broken, it shall be promptly repaired.

This Privy MUST be abandoned when Sewer is accessible.

By order of the
Board of Health

**THESE RULES
WILL BE STRICTLY
ENFORCED BY
THE DIVISION OF
SANITATION**

FOR FURTHER
INFORMATION CALL
AT THE
Division of Sanitation
615 CITY HALL

FLY SCREEN
DOOR SPRING
HINGED SELF CLOSING COVER
SELF CLOSING DOOR
BLOCK
BOX FOR UNSLACKED LIME
PRIVY WELL

THIS CARD MUST NOT BE REMOVED OR DEFACED

IN FIGHTING DISEASE a society reveals its knowledge, its beliefs, and its communal priorities. Different diseases, however, pose different sorts of biological and thus social problems—and each demands appropriate public health responses. The contrasting histories of diphtheria, tuberculosis, and influenza illustrate this diversity.

DIPHTHERIA

IN LATE-NINETEENTH-century urban America it was the young who suffered disproportionately from infectious disease. Children under the age of one died most frequently of gastrointestinal diseases, often caused by impure milk or water. Others were felled by typhoid, scarlet fever, whooping cough, and measles.

Diphtheria was one of the most fatal of the infectious bacterial diseases. Largely a disease of childhood, it was erratically endemic in large cities and occasionally flared into epidemic outbreaks. Easily spread by personal contact and by contaminated milk (prior to the use of pasteurization), its appearance provoked enormous alarm and, ultimately, effective precautions.

The diphtheria bacillus caused an inflammation of the throat and created a membrane over the air passages. It also produced a deadly systemic toxin that could cause paralysis of the heart and nervous system. In the late nineteenth century, treatment of diphtheria consisted of tracheotomy—opening a passage directly into the throat to allow a patient to breathe—and later, intubation, the insertion of a breathing tube in the throat. Intubation was an improvement, but mortality rates remained high. Such symptomatic relief could have little effect on the toxin already active in the patient's blood stream. In the twentieth century, however, new methods of diagnosis, using throat cultures, and new forms of treatment, using antitoxin, seem to have gradually lowered case fatality rates.

Some of the greatest and earliest triumphs of laboratory bacteriology came in the conquest of diphtheria, and its history is an illustration of the importance of laboratory findings to public health. Identification of the bacillus made it possible to perform throat cultures on those suspected of having an infection, including those who appeared healthy but carried the disease. More important, an antitoxin (conferring passive immunity), which became available after 1894, offered the hope of intervening in an ongoing case and lessened the need for surgical intervention. By 1913 physicians were able to confer active immunity by administering a combination of the toxin and an antitoxin. In 1923 a toxoid preparation, in which the immunizing property was preserved but the toxic potential removed, became available.

Despite the availability of prophylactic vaccination, there continued to be diphtheria outbreaks among those who had not been immunized. In these instances public health measures focused on preventing the further spread of the disease by quarantining and vaccinating infected persons and their contacts (whether or not they displayed symptoms) and by disinfecting household items and other goods capable of spreading the bacillus. Eventually the emphasis shifted from treatment to prevention. The Board of Health recommended that all young children be immunized and made the procedure widely available in clinics and in private medical practice. The board also advocated mandatory vaccination of children entering school.

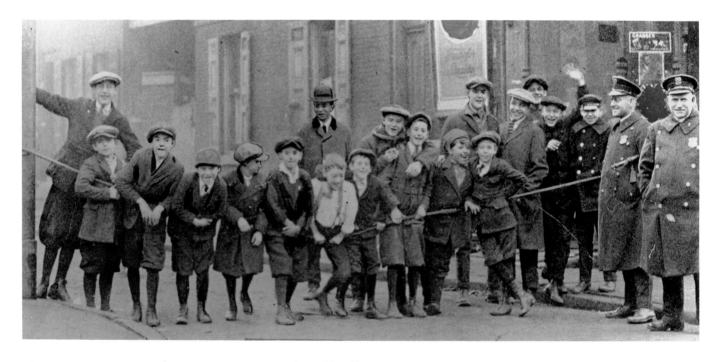

145.

Diphtheria quarantine.
Temple University Urban Archives.

AFTER DIPHTHERIA CASES were identified the city health department took quick action. Here a neighborhood has been quarantined—a rope is stretched across the street. But the crowd of young children chatting with the police officers suggests the limitations of such measures.

In 1926, PHILADELPHIA inaugurated an annual diphtheria immunization campaign. During a three-week period in June, the procedure was offered free to children between the ages of nine months and six years at the city's health centers and at public and parochial schools. Young children receiving their immunizations are pictured here.

Initially the program offered three injections of toxin antitoxin, but in 1935 it was replaced by a single injection of toxoid. The campaign was successful; between 1930 and 1934 Philadelphia had the lowest death rates from diphtheria of any major American city.

146.

Diphtheria immunization. *Temple University Urban Archives.*

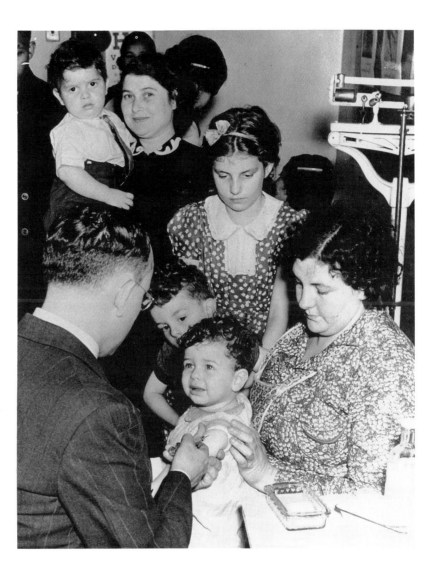

TUBERCULOSIS DISABLED AND killed more Philadelphians than any other nineteenth-century disease. In the 1870s and 1880s over two thousand citizens died each year from what was then called the "white plague." A chronic infection transmitted by airborne droplets and most often sited in the lung, tuberculosis afflicted those in the prime of life. Racked with fever, breathless, in pain, coughing and spitting blood, losing weight, its victims seemed to be consumed by their illness, so much so that the disease was popularly known as consumption.

The bacillus causing tuberculosis was discovered by Robert Koch in 1882, but effective treatments remained unavailable until the development of appropriate chemotherapy in the 1950s. Ironically, the "cure" came well after incidence of the disease had declined dramatically. Individual susceptibility with its reflection of diet and other environmental factors probably explained both the decline—and in all likelihood the original prevalence—of this omnipresent killer.

Treatment, control, and prevention were the watchwords in the early-twentieth-century fight against tuberculosis. Treatment, in the era before chemotherapy, consisted largely of a regimen of rest, a rich diet, fresh air, and sunshine. To control the spread of disease, public health officials advocated case registration and the isolation of those who seemed likely to infect others.

It had long been recognized that the poor suffered the highest rates of infection, and this in turn led to calls for effective health education in distressed neighborhoods and for improvements in living standards. But if the poor suffered disproportionately from this disease, no one was immune. Many physicians and nurses who were exposed eventually succumbed to the disease, and others lost years of their lives as they attempted to recover from infection. (Many leaders in the public fight against tuberculosis were recovered consumptives themselves.)

The fight against tuberculosis occurred in the community and in the legislature as well as at the bedside. Professionals and lay persons united in 1892 to found the Pennsylvania Tuberculosis Society. The society sponsored several exhibitions to educate the public in regards to tuberculosis prevention, worked with unions and other advocates of industrial hygiene to promote healthier working conditions, and fought on the state level for legislation and funding. Although rates of infection fell by the 1940s, the disease remained the seventh leading cause of death nationally, and the biggest killer of men and women between the ages of 20 and 45.

The frightening toll taken by tuberculosis and the number of volunteers and professionals who enlisted in the battle against it ensured a rich photographic heritage. Most of the images show the degree to which fresh air was seen as the best, if also a limited, intervention. At the same time these pictures present us with a view of a developing public health infrastructure that incorporated activities in hospitals, sanatoriums, clinics, schools, voluntary agencies, and state and local government, as well as in the community at large.

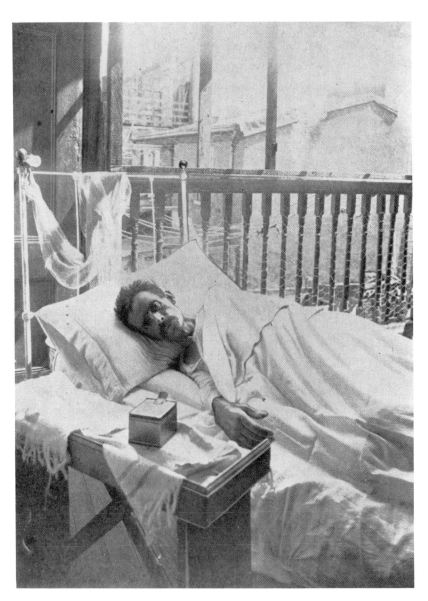

EXPOSURE TO THE fresh air, in winter and in summer, was a fundamental aspect of tuberculosis treatment before effective drugs became available. The wealthy could afford to seek the ideal climate and take their treatment in private sanitoriums. The poor too sought fresh air, and found it on tenement roofs, on porches, and in tents on hospital grounds.

The man resting on his tenement roof in this image from 1909 was a patient of the Philadelphia Visiting Nurse Society. He exhibits the emaciation characteristic of tuberculosis; further evidence of his condition is the spit cup on the table. The use of a spit cup and the disposal of its contents as well as other methods for preventing the infection of others (such as control over coughing) were some of the key personal hygiene lessons taught by visiting nurses.

147.

Man with spit cup.
Center for the Study of the History of Nursing, School of Nursing, University of Pennsylvania.

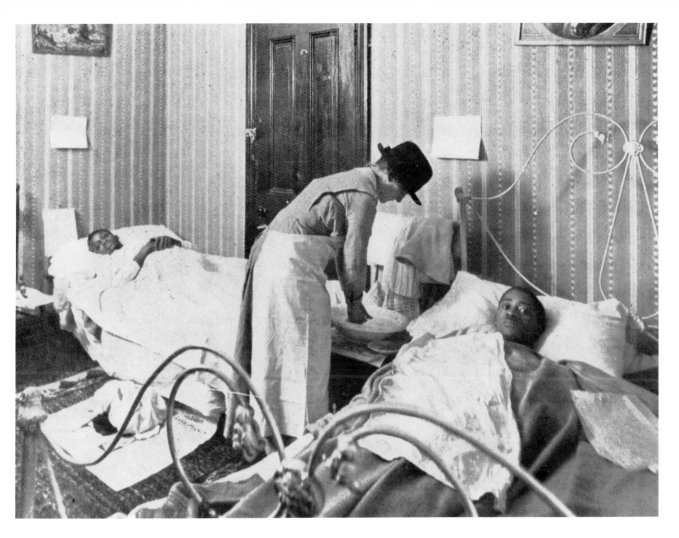

This image, printed in the 1916 annual report of the Visiting Nurse Society, bore the hopeful caption "Through the Service and Instruction of their Visiting Nurse, These Two Boys, the Principal Support of their Mother, May Recover and Be Able to Work Again." Tempering the report's optimism was the knowledge that tuberculosis was taking a severe toll in Philadelphia's black community. In 1915 the death rate from tuberculosis for the city's white population stood at 146 per 100,000 while for black citizens the rate was 388 per 100,000.

148.

Two tuberculous boys being visited by nurse. *Center for the Study of the History of Nursing, University of Pennsylvania.*

149.

Tuberculous men on
rooftop.
*Historical Collections,
College of Physicians of
Philadelphia.*

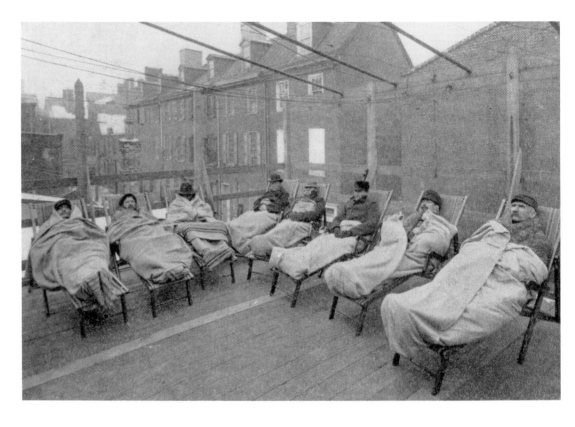

THE FIRST PRIVATE institution in Pennsylvania devoted to the care of consumptives was the House
of Mercy, established by the Philadelphia Protes-
tant Episcopal City Mission in 1876. Later the
same organization would open a home for female
consumptives in Chestnut Hill. Male residents
of the House of Mercy are shown here on the
"roof-garden."

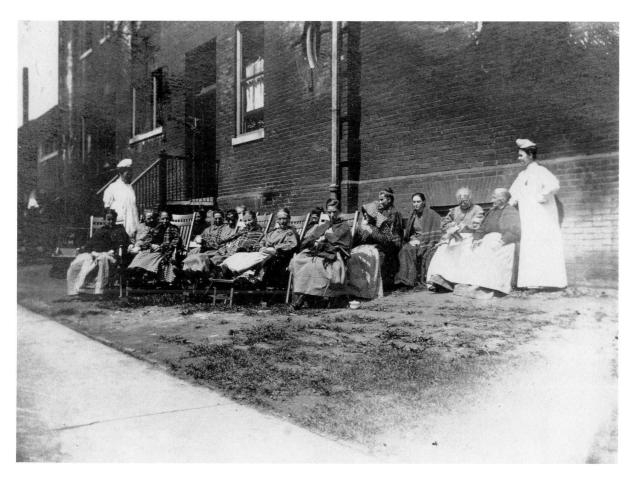

BEFORE AND AFTER the development of special
institutions for consumptives, poor patients with
tuberculosis received care at the Philadelphia
General Hospital. Until 1903, when special pavilions were built, the consumptive often mingled
with other patients in the surgical, medical, and
insane departments, a practice that undoubtedly
helped spread the disease. This image, from 1904,
shows patients outside the newly constructed
building for tuberculous women.

150.

Tuberculosis building,
Philadelphia General
Hospital.
*Historical Collections,
College of Physicians of
Philadelphia.*

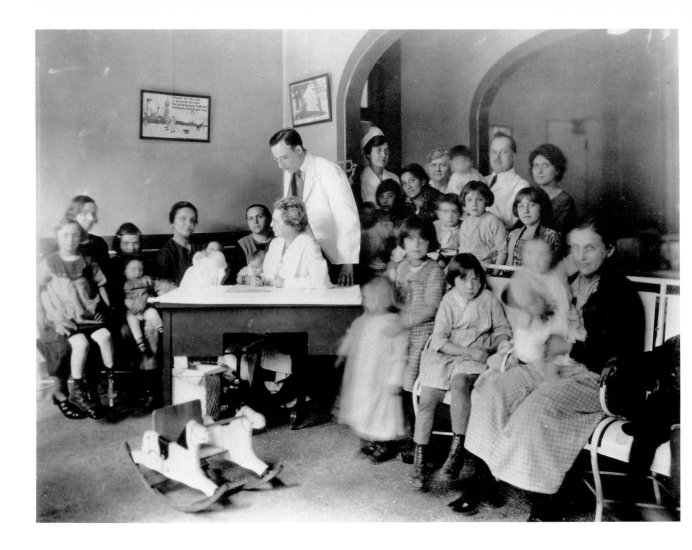

151.

Phipps Institute.
University of Pennsyl-
vania Archives.

THE PHIPPS INSTITUTE for the Study, Treatment
and Prevention of Tuberculosis opened in 1903
and became part of the University of Pennsylvania
in 1910. It included physicians' offices, a dispensary, inpatient wards, a laboratory, and a training
school for nurses. This image shows what is evi-
dently a children's clinic. The educational poster
on the wall reads "Please let me ask, If anyone
knows, You should keep your mouth shut, And
breathe through your nose."

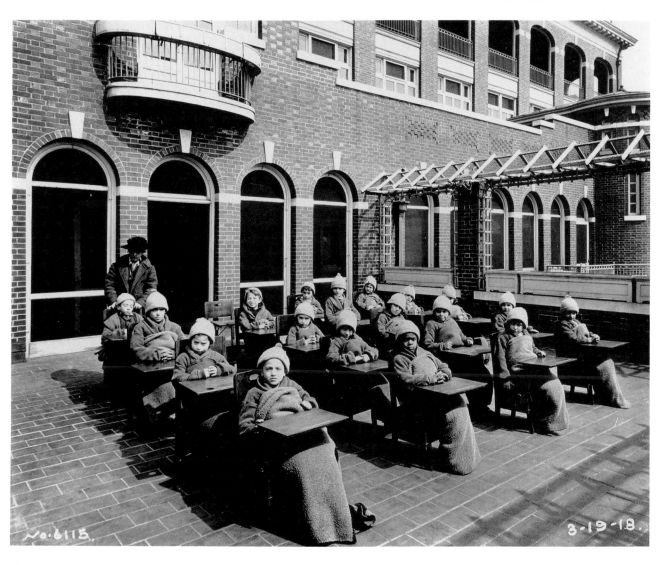

FOR YOUNGSTERS WITH mild cases of tuberculosis, exposed to the disease at home, or merely wan and sickly in appearance, the City of Philadelphia established open-air schools in 1911. While not necessarily effective in either treating or preventing the disease, the schools were an indication of the community's fear of tuberculosis. In this 1918 public school photograph a group of youngsters seem to be waiting for their lesson to begin.

152.

Outdoor school.
Temple University Urban Archives.

INFLUENZA

THE INFLUENZA PANDEMIC of 1918 killed an estimated 22 million worldwide; approximately half a million Americans succumbed to the disease in a ten-month period. An estimated 150,000 Philadelphians fell ill with the disease, of whom 12,687 succumbed to influenza or to the pneumonia that often accompanied it. This was a familiar disease in an unfamiliar—and unaccustomedly deadly—guise, and the responses to it were far different from those developed during the public's experience with tuberculosis. The influenza epidemic helped puncture a perhaps excessive medical confidence nurtured in a half-century of dramatic laboratory achievements.

Despite the drama of the 1918 influenza epidemic—or perhaps because of the fear it evoked—there are relatively few photographs recording its impact in Philadelphia. Those that do exist, however, are eloquent. This photograph, published in the *Philadelphia Evening Bulletin* in October 1918, shows an influenza victim, wrapped in a blanket, being escorted to the hospital by a police officer wearing a face mask.

153.

Influenza victim.
Temple University Urban Archives.

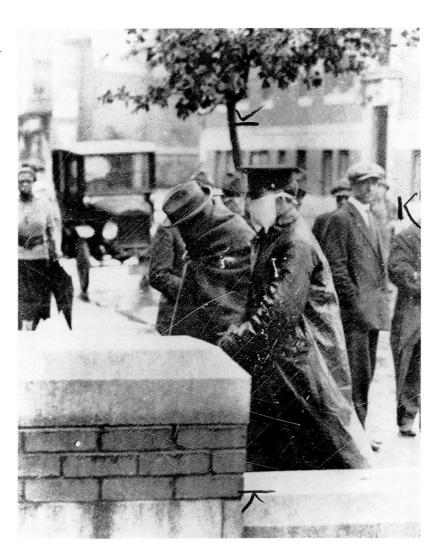

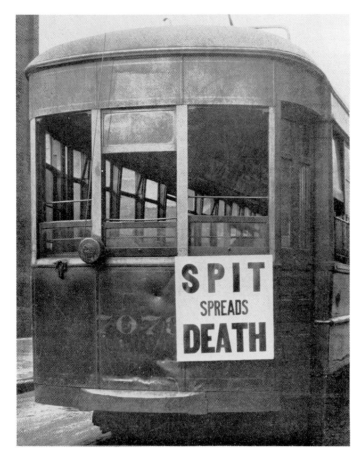

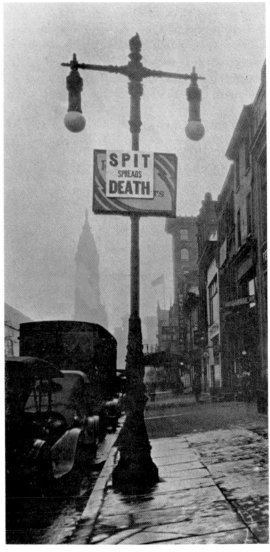

154.

"Spit spreads death" sign on trolley.
Temple University Urban Archives.

155.

"Spit spreads death" sign on streetlamp.
Temple University Urban Archives.

THIS PHOTOGRAPH COMES from a report issued by the health department and illustrates one of the publicity efforts undertaken to combat the epidemic. Soon after the disease arrived in Philadelphia the Board of Health began closing down public gathering places (including churches, schools, and saloons) and posting signs on public transportation. One warned, "To prevent the spread of Epidemic Influenza sneeze, cough or expectorate (if you must) in your handkerchief. You are in no danger if everyone heeds this warning." Others, attached to the outside of transit vehicles, ominously proclaimed "Spit Spreads Death." These measures proved insufficient to halt the spread of the disease; on a single day, October 15, 1918, 711 influenza and pneumonia deaths were recorded in the city.

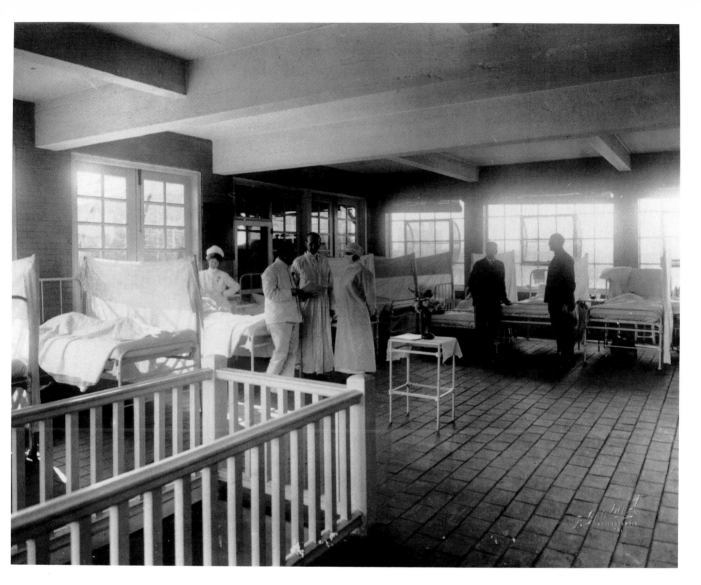

MEDICAL PROFESSIONALS WERE overwhelmed by the epidemic. With 1,000 physicians and 900 nurses absent on military duty, reinforcements were needed. Juniors and seniors from the city's medical colleges (which closed during the epidemic) attended patients lacking family physicians. Hospitals too were overwhelmed and ten facilities were opened in temporary locations such as clubs and churches. This photograph shows the influenza ward of Samaritan Hospital, which was affiliated with Temple University Medical School.

156.

Influenza ward, Samaritan Hospital. *Historical Society of Pennsylvania.*

Health Workers in the Community

Visiting Nurses

THE DEVELOPMENT OF public health nursing in the late nineteenth century was part of a larger effort by social reformers to respond to urban poverty. Many Philadelphians suffered from illnesses linked to poor nutrition, housing, and sanitation. To combat both the immediate reality of sickness and the underlying and pathogenic consequences of poverty, public health nurses combined care of the sick in their homes with instruction in health and hygiene. Visiting nurses worked for municipalities as well as for private voluntary agencies. Among their special concerns were efforts to improve maternal and child health, home care for the victims of tuberculosis, nursing in industry and public schools, and disaster relief through the Red Cross.

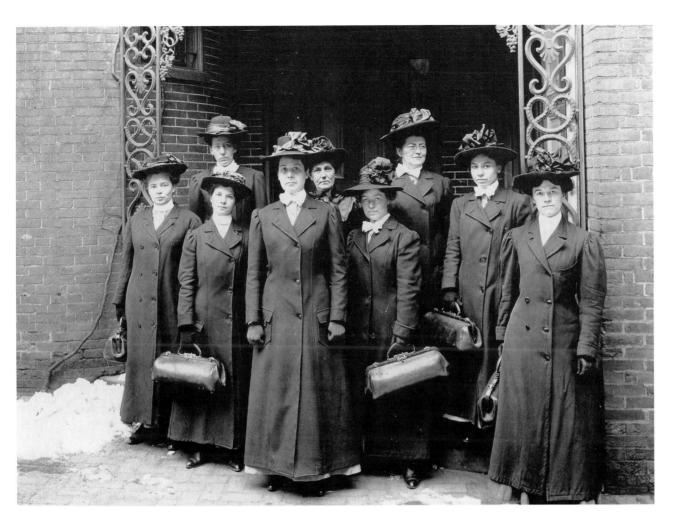

In a 1909 staff portrait of the Visiting Nurse Society of Philadelphia the nurses appear to be a formidable group. Their clothes indicate the social and often ethnic gap that separated the highly educated and predominantly native-born nurses from their tenement clients.

157.

Staff portrait, Visiting Nurse Society.
Center for the Study of the History of Nursing, School of Nursing, University of Pennsylvania.

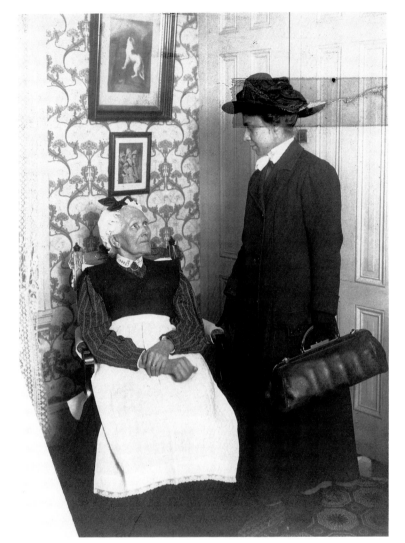

CARE OF BEDRIDDEN, chronically ill, or aged patients was just one of the many duties undertaken by visiting nurses. Two photographs of nurses attending elderly patients are posed to underline the nurses' status as skilled professionals.

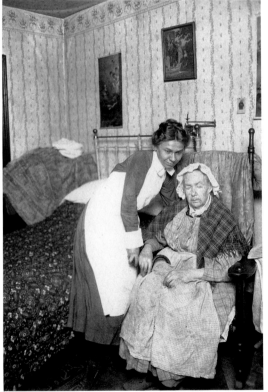

158.

Nurse visiting elderly patient.
Center for the Study of the History of Nursing, School of Nursing, University of Pennsylvania.

159.

Nurse with elderly patient.
Center for the Study of the History of Nursing, School of Nursing, University of Pennsylvania.

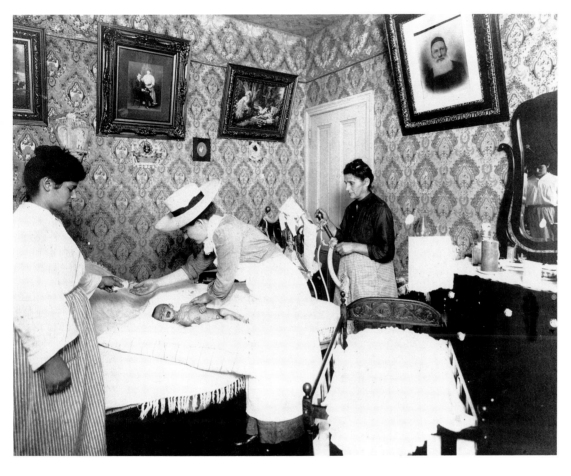

160.

Nurse in hat with new-
born and women.
*Center for the Study of
the History of Nursing,
School of Nursing, Uni-
versity of Pennsylvania.*

CARE OF NEWBORN and sick infants was one of
the primary duties of the public health nurse.
Philadelphia's infant mortality rate, like that of
other cities, was high, particularly in poor immigrant and non-white neighborhoods. The three
images on these pages displaying the work of
public health nurses also offer fascinating
glimpses into the rooms in which some Philadelphians bore, and reared, their children.

161.

Nurse with newborn and women.
Center for the Study of the History of Nursing, School of Nursing, University of Pennsylvania.

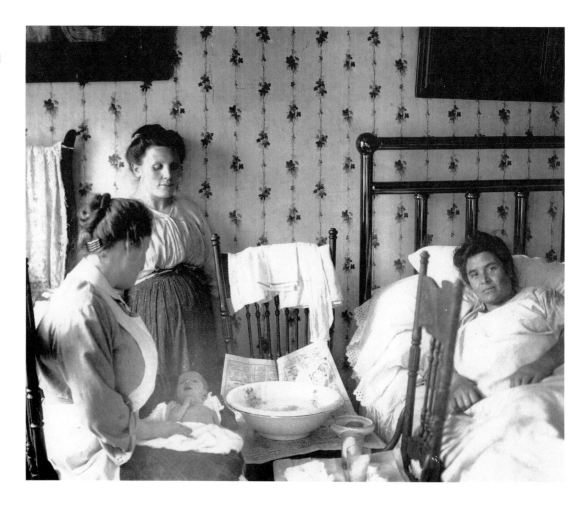

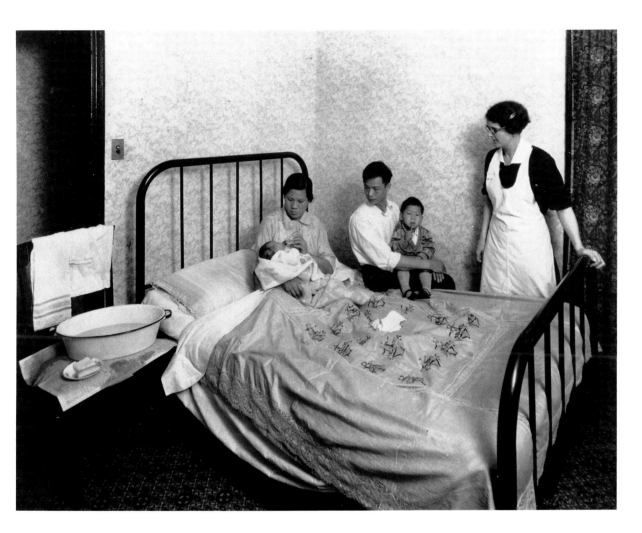

162.

Nurse with Asian family and newborn.
Center for the Study of the History of Nursing, School of Nursing, University of Pennsylvania.

AT THE TURN of the century, midwives delivered the majority of babies born in Philadelphia's immigrant neighborhoods. In the early twentieth century, midwives were supervised by the Bureau of Medical Education and Licensure, which hired female physicians able to "speak the various languages necessary in midwife work." By the Depression years, however, the practice of midwifery was in decline. The medicalization of childbirth is one explanation. Some women believed that medically supervised births, whether at home or in the hospital, offered advantages in safety and pain relief. But another explanation for this transition, offered by the midwives themselves, was economic. Women could receive free maternity care at the Philadelphia Lying-In Hospital and other charitable institutions; they would never think of asking the neighborhood midwife to work without compensation.

Midwives were never photographed "on the job." Only family photographs show us these early-twentieth century health providers.

SALAMEA MACKIEWICZ, a midwife trained in Poland, emigrated to the United States in the late nineteenth century. She practiced midwifery in the Bridesburgh-Tacony area until the late 1930s.

Anna Carastro received her midwife training at the University of Catonia in Sicily and practiced midwifery in Italy for three years. She emigrated with her husband to the United States and practiced midwifery in South Philadelphia from 1924 until 1940, when her practice declined. She then opened a licensed private day nursery.

Maria Straka, an immigrant from Austria, learned her trade by apprenticeship. She lived in the Grey's Ferry area, where she could serve other Austrian immigrants, and in order to expand her practice learned seven other languages, including Polish, Russian, Italian, and Yiddish. She had a busy practice of between twelve and sixteen births each month and between 1910 and 1938 registered over 1,300 births. Like Anna Carastro, she stopped practicing because it was no longer lucrative.

Rebecca Gorodetzer, a Russian Jewish immigrant from Kiev, was a university-trained midwife who emigrated to the United States in the early twentieth century. She practiced among Russian Jewish immigrants in the Moyamensing area of Philadelphia until the late 1930s.

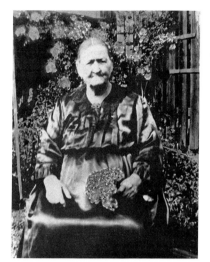
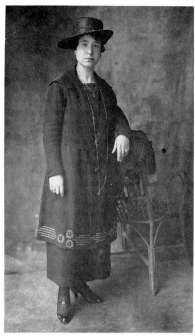
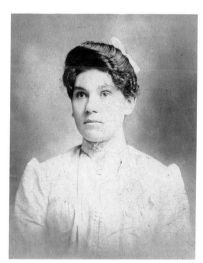
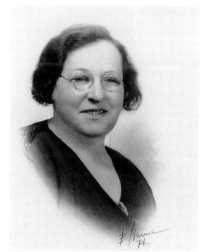

163.

Salamea Mackiewicz.
Privately held.

164.

Anna Carastro.
Privately held.

165.

Maria Straka.
Privately held.

166.

Rebecca Gorodetzer.
Privately held.

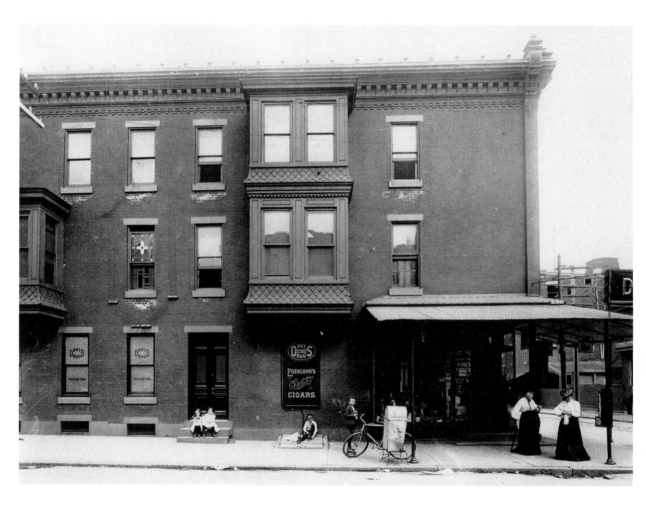

167.

Exterior of pharmacy.
*City Archives of
Philadelphia.*

THE COMMUNITY PHARMACY served those filling prescriptions from physicians or selecting over-the-counter medications; in a good many instances proprietor pharmacists served as informal general practitioners for their neighbors.

The first image shows the exterior of a drug store located on the northeast corner of 7th and Oxford Streets in 1904. The second photograph shows the interior of a neighborhood pharmacy.

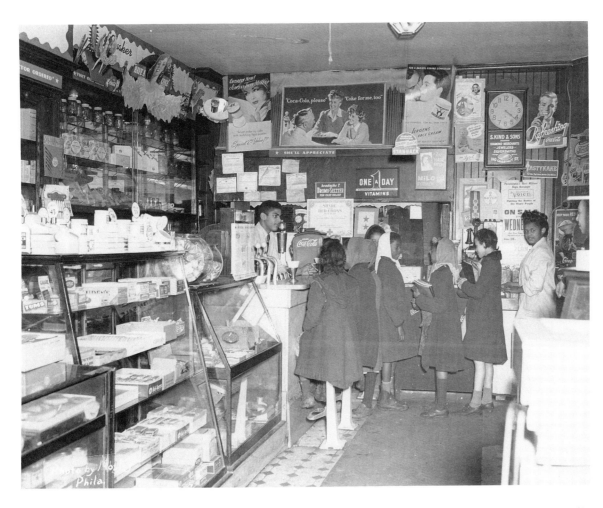

168.

Interior of pharmacy.
*Charles L. Blockson
Afro-American Collec-
tion, Temple University.*

169.

Office of S. Weir Mitchell.
Historical Collections, College of Physicians of Philadelphia.

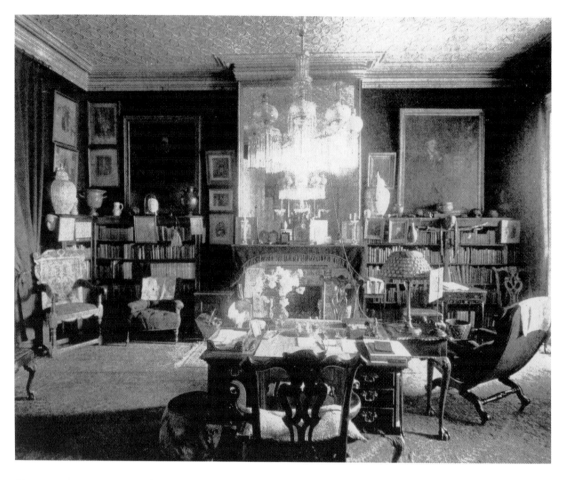

DESPITE THE PLETHORA of images of hospital operating rooms, clinics, wards, and laboratories, the most common encounter between doctor and patient was that which took place in the physician's office. While the hospital became the place in which acute illnesses were diagnosed and treated, the private office continued to be the place where patients presented practitioners with the majority of their complaints—from minor aches and pains to life-threatening diseases.

Physicians' consulting rooms ranged from the simple and unadorned office of the neighborhood general practitioner to the more elaborate suites of the city's elite consultants. This image records the consulting room of S. Weir Mitchell (1830–1913), one of America's most prominent neurologists.

DR. LEMUEL T. SEWELL (?1889–1973) and his son Dr. Edward M. Sewell (?1923–1990) shown here served the Philadelphia community for many decades. L. T. Sewell graduated from Hahnemann Medical College in 1911; he was chief of the obstetrical service and president of the medical staff of Mercy Hospital. E. M. Sewell graduated from the University of Pennsylvania School of Medicine and was a pediatric resident at the Children's Hospital of Philadelphia. He held a number of teaching and administrative positions in the city, and served as president of the national American Lung Association.

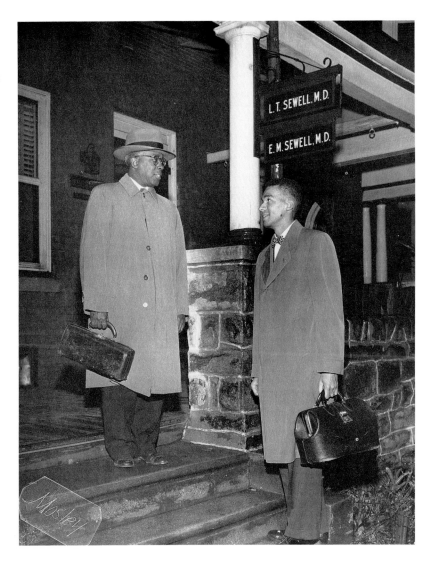

170.

Sewells.
Charles L. Blockson Afro-American Collection, Temple University.

Bibliography

Abrahams, Harold J. *Extinct Medical Schools of Nineteenth-Century Philadelphia.* Philadelphia: University of Pennsylvania Press, 1966.

Albert, Daniel M. and Harold G. Scheie. *A History of Ophthalmology at the University of Pennsylvania.* Springfield, Ill.: Thomas, 1965.

———. "Ophthalmology at the University of Pennsylvania: A Chronology." *Transactions and Studies of the College of Physicians of Philadelphia* 4th ser. 34 (1966/67): 83–88.

Alewitz, Sam. "Sanitation and Public Health: Philadelphia, 1870–1900." Ph.D. Dissertation, Case Western Reserve University, 1981.

Alexander, John K. "Institutional Imperialism and the Sick Poor in Late-Eighteenth-Century Philadelphia: The House of Employment versus the Pennsylvania Hospital." *Pennsylvania History* 51 (1984): 101–117.

Alsop, Gulielma Fell. *History of the Woman's Medical College, Philadelphia, Pennsylvania, 1850–1950.* Philadelphia: Lippincott, 1950.

Baatz, Simon. "'A Very Diffused Disposition': Dissecting Schools in Philadelphia, 1823–1825." *Pennsylvania Magazine of History and Biography* 108 (1984): 203–217.

Baker, Samuel L. "Physician Licensure Laws in the United States, 1865–1915." *Journal of the History of Medicine and Allied Sciences* 39 (April 1984): 173–197.

Bauer, Edward Louis. *Doctors Made in America.* Philadelphia: Lippincott, 1963.

Becker, Howard S. "Do Photographs Tell the Truth?" *Afterimage* (1978): 9–13.

Bell, Whitfield J. *The College of Physicians of Philadelphia: A Bicentennial History.* Canton, Mass.: Science History Publications, 1987.

Bliss, Arthur Ames. *Blockley Days: Memories and Impressions of a Resident Physician, 1883–1884.* Springfield, Mass.: Privately printed, 1916.

Bond, Earl Danforth. *Dr. Kirkbride and His Mental Hospital.* Philadelphia: Lippincott, 1947.

Bradford, Thomas Lindsay. *History of the Homeopathic Medical College of Pennsylvania: The Hahnemann Medical College and Hospital of Philadelphia.* Philadelphia: Boericke & Tafel, 1898.

Brecher, Edward M. *The Rays: A History of Radiology in the United States and Canada.* Baltimore: Williams & Wilkins, 1969.

Bromer, Ralph S. "The History of Radiology in Philadelphia: The History of the Philadelphia Roentgen Ray Society, Part II: 1920–1954." *American Journal of Roentgenology* 75 (1956): 23–29.

Buhler-Wilkerson, Karen. "False Dawn: The Rise and Decline of Public Health Nursing, 1900–1930." Ph.D. dissertation, University of Pennsylvania, 1984.

———, ed. *Nursing and the Public's Health: An Anthology of Sources.* New York: Garland, 1989.

Burns, Stanley. *Early Medical Photography in America.* New York: Burns Archive, 1983.

Byrnes, Mary Beth. *Celebrating One Hundred Years of Excellence in Nursing Education: Presbyterian School of Nursing, 1887–1987.* Philadelphia: Presbyterian School of Nursing, 1987.

Carson, Joseph. *History of the Medical Department of the University of Pennsylvania, from Its Foundation in 1765: With Sketches of the Lives of Deceased Professors.* Philadelphia: Lindsay & Blakiston, 1869.

Casterline, Gail Farr. "St. Joseph's and St. Mary's: The Origins of Catholic Hospitals in Philadelphia." *Pennsylvania Magazine of History and Biography* 108 (1984): 289–314.

Caulfield, Ernest. "The General State of American Pediatrics in 1855, with Particular Reference to Philadelphia." *Pediatrics* 19 (1957): 456–461.

Chance, Burton. "Ophthalmology in Philadelphia in the Early 1890s." *Transactions and Studies of the College of Physicians of Philadelphia* 4th ser. 11 (1943): 77–81.

Cherry, Charles L. "Friends' Asylum, Morgan Hinchman, and Moral Insanity." *Quaker History* 67 (1978): 20–34.

Cheyney, Edward Potts. *History of the University of Pennsylvania, 1740–1940.* Philadelphia: University of Pennsylvania Press, 1940.

Condran, Gretchen A. and Rose A. Cheney. "Mortality Trends in Philadelphia: Age- and Cause-Specific Death Rates, 1870–1930." *Demography* 19 (1982): 97–123.

Condran, Gretchen A., Henry Williams, and Rose A. Cheney. "The Decline in Mortality in Philadelphia from 1870 to 1930: The Role of Municipal Services." *Pennsylvania Magazine of History and Biography* 108 (1984): 153–177.

Cone, Thomas E., Jr. "Purulent Ophthalmia in the Children's Asylum of the Philadelphia Almshouse in 1836." *Pediatrics* 69 (1982): 480.

Corner, Betsy Copping. *William Shippen, Jr.: Pioneer in American Medical Education.* Philadelphia: American Philosophical Society, 1951.

Corner, George Washington. *Two Centuries of Medicine: A History of the School of Medicine, University of Pennsylvania.* Philadelphia: Lippincott, 1965.

Cronje, Gillian. "Tuberculosis and Mortality Decline in England and Wales, 1851–1900." In Robert Wood and John Woodward, eds., *Urban Disease and Mortality in Nineteenth-Century England.* London and New York: St. Martin's, 1984.

Croskey, John Walsh, comp. *History of Blockley: A History of the Philadelphia General Hospital from Its Inception, 1731–1928.* Philadelphia: Davis, 1929.

Cushing, Harvey W. *The Life of Sir William Osler.* Oxford: Clarendon, 1925.

Cutler, William W. III and Howard Gillette Jr., eds. *The Divided Metropolis: Social and Spatial Dimensions of Philadelphia, 1800–1975.* Westport, Conn.: Greenwood, 1980.

Davidson, James West and Lytle, Mark Hamilton. "The Mirror With a Memory." In Davidson and Lytle, *After the Fact: The Art of Historical Detection*, pp. 205–231. New York: Knopf, 1982.

Davis, Allen F. and Mark H. Haller, eds. *The Peoples of Philadelphia: A History of Ethnic Groups and Lower-Class Life, 1790–1840*. Philadelphia: Temple University Press, 1973.

Davis, Nathan Smith. *Contributions to the History of Medical Education and Medical Institutions in the United States of America, 1776–1876*. Washington, D.C.: U.S. Government Printing Office, 1877.

Department of Public Health and Charities of the City of Philadelphia. *What the Health Department Has Done to Curb the Epidemic of Influenza. Monthly Bulletin* 3 (10/11) (Oct.–Nov. 1918).

Department of Public Health. *Annual Statistical Report, 1980. Division of Health Program Analysis*. Philadelphia: City of Philadelphia, n.d.

Deutsch, Albert. *The Mentally Ill in America: A History of Their Care and Treatment from Colonial Times*. New York: Doubleday, Doran, 1937.

Donatucci, Craig F. "In Anticipation of Flexner." *Transactions and Studies of the College of Physicians of Philadelphia* 4th ser. 45 (1978): 280–290.

Dowdall, George W., and Janet Golden. "Photographs as Data: An Analysis of Images from a Mental Hospital." *Qualitative Sociology* 12 (1989): 183–213.

Downie, Robert W. "Pennsylvania Hospital Admissions, 1751–1850: A Survey." *Transactions and Studies of the College of Physicians of Philadelphia* 4th ser. 32 (1964/65): 20–35.

Eckenhoff, James Edward. *Anesthesia from Colonial Times: A History of Anesthesia at the University of Pennsylvania*. Philadelphia: Lippincott, 1966.

Emerson, Haven, et al. *Philadelphia Health and Hospital Survey, 1929*. Philadelphia: Philadelphia Health and Hospital Survey Committee, 1930.

Flexner, Abraham. *Medical Education in the United States and Canada: A Report to the Carnegie Foundation for the Advancement of Teaching*. New York: The Carnegie Foundation for the Advancement of Teaching, 1910.

Fox, Daniel M. and Christopher Lawrence. *Photographing Medicine: Images and Power in Britain and America Since 1840*. Westport, Conn. and London: Greenwood, 1988.

Fox, Daniel M. and James S. Terry. "Photography and the Self-Image of American Physicians." *Bulletin of the History of Medicine* 52 (1978): 435–457.

Frese, Carl. *A Short History and Description of the German Hospital, Philadelphia, Pennsylvania*. 2nd ed., rev. A.D. Whiting, Philadelphia: Girard Printing House, 1895.

Friedman, Emily. "The Demise of Philadelphia General, An Instructive Case" and subsequent correspondence. *Journal of the American Medical Association* 257 (1978): 1571–1572, 1574–1575; 258 (1987): 327.

Friedman, Reuben. *A History of Dermatology in Philadelphia. Including a Biography of Louis A. Duhring, Father of Dermatology in Philadelphia*. Fort Pierce Beach, Fla.: Froben, 1955.

Gamble, Vanessa. *The Black Community Hospital: Contemporary Dilemmas in Historical Perspective*. New York: Garland, 1989.

————. *Germs Have No Color Line: Blacks and American Medicine, 1900–1945. An Anthology of Sources*. New York: Garland, 1989.

————. "The Negro Hospital Renaissance: The Black Hospital Movement, 1920–1940." Ph.D. dissertation, University of Pennsylvania, 1987.

Gayley, James F. *A History of the Jefferson Medical College of Philadelphia*. Philadelphia: J. M. Wilson, 1858.

Gilman, Sander. *Disease and Representation: Images of Illness from Madness to AIDS*. Ithaca, N.Y.: Cornell University Press, 1988.

————. *Seeing the Insane*. New York: Wiley, 1982.

Golden, Janet, ed. *Infant Asylums and Children's Hospitals: Medical Dilemmas and Developments, 1850–1920: An Anthology of Sources*. New York: Garland, 1989.

Griscom, Mary W. "History of the Woman's Hospital of Philadelphia: On Adventure Bound, 1861–1934." *Medical Woman's Journal* 41 (Nov. 1934): 291–295 and 41 (Dec. 1934): 318–325.

Gross, Samuel David. *Autobiography, with Sketches of His Contemporaries, Edited by His Sons*. 2 vols. Philadelphia: Barrie, 1887.

Hales, Peter B. *Silver Cities: The Photography of American Urbanization, 1839–1915*. Philadelphia: Temple University Press, 1984.

Harris, Neil. "Iconography and Intellectual History: The Half-Tone Effect." In John Higham and Paul K. Conkin, eds., *New Directions in American Intellectual History*, pp. 196–211. Baltimore: Johns Hopkins University Press, 1979.

Henry, Frederick P., ed. *Founders' Week Memorial Volume: Containing an Account of the 225th Anniversary of the Founding of the City of Philadelphia, and Histories of Its Principal Scientific Institutions, Medical Colleges, Hospitals, etc.* Philadelphia: City of Philadelphia, 1909.

Hepburn, Joseph Samuel. "Pioneer Biochemical Researches at the University of Pennsylvania." *Journal of the Franklin Institute* 261 (6) (June 1956): 637–648.

Hershberg, Theodore, ed. *Philadelphia: Work, Space, Family, and Group Experience in the Nineteenth Century*. New York: Oxford University Press, 1981.

Hine, Darlene Clark. *Black Women in White: Racial Conflict and Cooperation in the Nursing Profession, 1890–1950*. Bloomington: Indiana University Press, 1989.

Howell, Joel D. "Early Use of X-ray Machines and Electrocardiographs at the Pennsylvania Hospital, 1897 through 1927." *Journal of the American Medical Association* 255 (1986): 2320–2323.

————. "Machines' Meanings: British and American Use of Medical Technology, 1890–1930." Ph.D. dissertation, University of Pennsylvania, 1987.

————. *Technology and American Medical Practice. 1880–1930: An Anthology of Sources*. New York: Garland, 1989.

Hunter, Robert J., "Dedication of the Osler Memorial Building of the Philadelphia General Hospital, 'Old Blockley' June 8, 1940: How an Idea Grew into a Reality." *Bulletin of the History of Medicine* 10 (1941): 57–104.

————. *The Origin of the Philadelphia General Hospital, Blockley Division.* Philadelphia: Published by the author, 1955. Reprint with some revisions of "The Origin of the Philadelphia General Hospital," *Pennsylvania Magazine of History and Biography* 57 (1933): 32–57.

Jacobs, Maurice S., ed. *The Northern Medical Association of Philadelphia.* Philadelphia: The Association, 1946.

Jenkins, Reese V. *Images and Enterprise: Technology and the American Photographic Industry, 1839–1925* Baltimore: Johns Hopkins University Press, 1975.

Kaiser, Robert M., Sandra L. Chaff, and Steven J. Peitzman, "The Diary of Mary Theodora McGavran." *Pennsylvania Magazine of History and Biography* 108 (1984): 217–236.

Kalisch, Philip A. and Beatrice J. Kalisch. *The Advance of American Nursing.* 2nd ed. Boston: Little, Brown, 1986.

Kaufman, Martin. *American Medical Education: The Formative Years, 1765–1910.* Westport, Conn.: Greenwood, 1976.

————. *Homeopathy in America: The Rise and Fall of a Medical Heresy.* Baltimore: Johns Hopkins University Press, 1971.

King, William H., ed. *History of Homeopathy and its Institutions in America.* 4 vols. New York: Lewis, 1905.

Kohler, Robert E. *From Medical Chemistry to Biochemistry: The Making of a Biomedical Discipline.* New York: Cambridge University Press, 1982.

Konkle, Burton A. *Standard History of the Medical Profession of Philadelphia.* 2nd ed., enlarged and corrected. New York: AMS, 1977.

Krumbhaar, Edward B. "The History of Pathology at the Philadelphia General Hospital." *Medical Life* 40 (1933): 162–177.

La Colonia Italiana di Filadelfia. Philadelphia: 1906.

Lawrence, Charles. *History of the Philadelphia Almshouses and Hospitals.* . . . Philadelphia: Published by the author, 1905.

Layne, George S. "Kirkbride-Langenheim Collaboration: Early Use of Photography in Psychiatric Treatment in Philadelphia." *Pennsylvania Magazine of History and Biography* 105 (1981): 182–202.

Leake, Eva S. "The Henry Phipps Institute: Recollections of a Foreign Research Fellow." *Transactions and Studies of the College of Physicians of Philadelphia* 5th ser. 5 (1981): 256–263.

Leavitt, Judith Walzer. *Brought to Bed: Childbearing in America, 1750–1950.* New York: Oxford University Press, 1986.

————. *The Healthiest City: Milwaukee and the Politics of Health Reform.* Princeton, N.J.: Princeton University Press, 1983.

Leavitt, Judith Walzer and Ronald L. Numbers. *Sickness and Health in America: Readings in the History of Medicine and Public Health.* 2nd ed., rev. Madison: University of Wisconsin Press, 1985.

Liebenau, Jonathan M. "Public Health and the Production and Use of Diphtheria

Antitoxin in Philadelphia." *Bulletin of the History of Medicine* 61 (1987): 216–236.

Lloyd, Mark Frazier. *A History of Caring for the Sick Since 1863*. Philadelphia: Germantown Hospital and Medical Center, 1981.

Long, Diana Elizabeth, and Janet Golden, eds. *The American General Hospital: Communities and Social Context*. Ithaca, N.Y.: Cornell University Press, 1989.

Ludmerer, Kenneth M. *Learning to Heal: The Development of American Medical Education*. New York: Basic Books, 1985.

Malin, William G. *Some Account of the Pennsylvania Hospital, Its Origin, Objects, and Present State*. Philadelphia: Kite, 1831.

Marshall, Clara. *Woman's Medical College of Pennsylvania: An Historical Outline*. Philadelphia: Blakiston, 1897.

McBride, David. "The Henry Phipps Institute, 1903–1937: Pioneering Tuberculosis Work with an Urban Minority." *Bulletin of the History of Medicine* 61 (1987): 78–97.

———. *Integrating the City of Medicine: Blacks in Philadelphia Health Care, 1910–1965*. Philadelphia: Temple University Press, 1989.

McCord, Colin and Harold Freeman. "Excess Mortality in Harlem." *New England Journal of Medicine* 322 (1990): 173–177.

McFarland, Joseph. "The Beginnings of Bacteriology in Philadelphia." *Bulletin of the Institute of the History of Medicine* 5 (1937): 148–198.

———. "The History of Nursing at the Blockley Hospital." *Medical Life* 40 (1933): 177–191.

McKeown, Thomas. *The Role of Medicine: Dream, Mirage, or Nemesis?* Princeton, N.J.: Princeton University Press, 1979.

Meigs, J. Forsyth. *History of the First Quarter of the Second Century of the Pennsylvania Hospital*. Philadelphia: Collins, 1877.

Melosh, Barbara. *The Physician's Hand: Work, Culture and Conflict in American Nursing*. Philadelphia: Temple University Press, 1982.

Metropolitan Life Insurance Co. *Your Rights and Duties Under the Health Laws in Philadelphia, Pa*. Philadelphia: The Company, 1929.

Meyerson, Martin, and Dilys Pegler Winegrad. *Gladly Learn and Gladly Teach: Franklin and His Heirs at the University of Pennsylvania, 1740–1976*. Philadelphia: University of Pennsylvania Press, 1976.

Middleton, William Snow. "Clinical Teaching in the Philadelphia Almshouse and Hospital." *Medical Life* 40 (1933): 207–255.

Miller, Albert G. *History of the German Hospital of the City of Philadelphia and Its Ex-resident Physicians*. Philadelphia: Lippincott, 1906.

Miller, Frederic M., Morris J. Vogel, and Allen F. Davis. *Philadelphia Stories: A Photographic History, 1920–1960*. Philadelphia: Temple University Press, 1988.

———. *Still Philadelphia: A Photographic History, 1890–1940*. Philadelphia: Temple University Press, 1983.

Miller, T. G. "The Development of Specialty Medical Clinics at the University of Pennsylvania Hospital." *Transactions and Studies of the College of Physicians of Philadelphia* 4th ser. 32 (1964/65): 104–108.

Mitchell, S. Weir. *Address to the Nurse-Graduates of the Philadelphia Orthopaedic Hospital and Infirmary for Nervous Diseases,* November 16, 1906. Philadelphia: n.p., 1906.

Morais, Herbert Montfort. *The History of the Negro in Medicine.* New York: Publishers Co., 1968.

Morantz-Sanchez, Regina Markell. *Sympathy and Science: Women Physicians in American Medicine.* New York: Oxford University Press, 1985.

Morman, Edward T. "Clinical Pathology in America, 1865–1915: Philadelphia as a Test Case." *Bulletin of the History of Medicine* 58 (1984): 198–214.

———. *Efficiency, Scientific Management, and Hospital Standardization: An Anthology of Sources.* New York: Garland, 1989.

———. "Guarding Against Impurities: The Philadelphia Lazaretto, 1854–1893." *Pennsylvania Magazine of History and Biography* 108 (1984): 131–151.

———. "Scientific Medicine Comes to Philadelphia: Public Health Transformed, 1854–1899." Ph.D. dissertation, University of Pennsylvania, 1986.

Morton, Thomas G. *The History of the Pennsylvania Hospital, 1751–1895.* Rev. ed. Philadelphia: Times Printing House, 1897.

Morton, Thomas G., and William Hunt. *Surgery in the Pennsylvania Hospital, Being an Epitome of the Practice of the Hospital Since 1756; Including Collations from the Surgical Notes, and an Account of the More Interesting Cases from 1873 to 1878; with Some Statistical Tables, with Papers by John B. Roberts and Frank Woodbury.* Philadelphia: Lippincott, 1880.

Newhall, Beaumont. *The History of Photography: From 1839 to the Present.* Rev. and enlarged ed. New York: Museum of Modern Art, 1982.

Norris, George W. *The Housing Problem in Philadelphia.* Philadelphia: McVey, 1913.

Norwood, William Fred. *Medical Education in the United States Before the Civil War.* Philadelphia: University of Pennsylvania Press, 1944.

O'Brien, Patricia. "'All a Woman's Life Can Bring': The Domestic Roots of Nursing in Philadelphia, 1830–1885." *Nursing Research* 36 (1) (Jan.–Feb. 1987): 12–17.

O'Hara, Leo J. *An Emerging Profession: Philadelphia Doctors, 1860–1900.* New York: Garland, 1989.

Packard, Francis Randolph. *History of Medicine in the United States.* 2 vols. New York: Hoeber, 1931.

———. *Some Account of the Pennsylvania Hospital from its First Rise to the Beginning of the Year 1938 . . . with a Continuation of the Account to the Year 1956 by Florence M. Greim.* 2nd pr. Philadelphia: Engle, 1957.

Peitzman, Steven J. "The Quiet Life of a Philadelphia Medical Woman: Mary Willits (1855–1902)." *Journal of the American Medical Women's Association* 34 (Dec. 1979): 443–460.

―――. "'Thoroughly Practical': America's Polyclinic Medical Schools." *Bulletin of the History of Medicine* 54 (1980): 166–187.

Penman, W. Robert. "William Goodell, M.D., and the Preston Retreat." *Transactions and Studies of the College of Physicians of Philadelphia* 4th ser. 40 (1972/73): 112–119.

Pepper, William. *Account of the Inauguration of the Hospital of the University of Pennsylvania.* Philadelphia: n.p., 1874.

Peterman, Cy. *The Seventy-Fifth Anniversary History of the Philadelphia College of Osteopathic Medicine.* Kutztown, Pa.: Kutztown Publishing Co., 1974.

Pfahler, George E. "The Early History of Roentgenology in Philadelphia: the History of the Philadelphia Roentgen Ray Society, 1905–1920, Part I, 1899–1920." *American Journal of Roentgenology* 75 (1956): 14–22.

Posey, William C., and Samuel Horton Brown. *The Wills Hospital of Philadelphia. The Influence of European and British Ophthalmology upon It, and the Part It Played in Developing Ophthalmology in America.* Philadelphia: Lippincott, 1931.

Radbill, Samuel X. "The Children's Hospital of Philadelphia." *Philadelphia Medicine* 70 (1974): 352–367.

―――. "The Philadelphia Medical Society, 1789–1868." *Transactions and Studies of the College of Physicians of Philadelphia* 4th ser. 20 (1952/53): 103–123.

―――. "Saint Christopher's Hospital of Philadelphia." *Philadelphia Medicine* 69 (1973): 277–287, 328–336.

―――. "A Short History of the Philadelphia County Medical Society." *Philadelphia Medicine* 81 (1965): 165–167.

Ravenel, Mazyck. *A Half Century of Public Health.* New York: American Public Health Association, 1921.

Reiser, Stanley Joel. *Medicine and the Reign of Technology.* New York: Cambridge University Press, 1978.

Reverby, Susan. *Ordered to Care: The Dilemma of American Nursing, 1850–1945.* New York: Cambridge University Press, 1987.

Reverby, Susan and David Rosner, eds. *Health Care in America: Essays in Social History.* Philadelphia: Temple University Press, 1979.

Riesman, David. "Clinical Teaching in America, with Some Remarks on Early Medical Schools." *Transactions and Studies of the College of Physicians of Philadelphia* 4th ser. 7 (1939): 89–110.

Rodegra, Heinz. "Zur Geschichte des Deutschen Hospitals in Philadelphia (U.S.A.)." *History of Hospitals* (Dusseldorf) 14 (1981/82): 179–190.

Rogers, Fred B. "Osler and Philadelphia." *Transactions and Studies of the College of Physicians of Philadelphia* 4th ser. 38 (1971/72): 118–123.

Rogers, Naomi. "The Proper Place of Homeopathy: Hahnemann Medical College and Hospital in an Age of Scientific Medicine." *Pennsylvania Magazine of History and Biography* 108 (1984): 179–201.

————. "Screen the Baby, Swat the Fly: Polio in the Northeastern United States, 1916." Ph.D. dissertation, University of Pennsylvania, 1986.

Rosen, George. "Early Medical Photography." *Ciba Symposium*, Aug.–Sept. 1942, pp. 1344–1355.

————. *A History of Public Health.* New York: MD Publications, 1958.

————. *Preventive Medicine in the United States, 1900–1975: Trends and Interpretations.* New York: Science History Publications, 1975.

Rosenberg, Charles E. "Between Two Worlds: American Medicine in 1879." In John Blake, ed. *Centennary of Index Medicus*, pp. 3–18. Washington, D.C.: U.S. Government Printing Office, 1980.

————. *The Care of Strangers: The Rise of America's Hospital System.* New York: Basic Books, 1987.

————. "From Almshouse to Hospital: The Shaping of Philadelphia General Hospital." *Milbank Memorial Fund Quarterly* 60 (1) (1982): 108–154.

————. "Social Class and Medical Care in Nineteenth-Century America: The Rise and Fall of the Dispensary." *Journal of the History of Medicine* 29 (1974): 32–54.

————. "What It Was Like to Be Sick in 1884." *American Heritage* 35 (1984): 22–31.

Rosner, David. *A Once Charitable Enterprise: Hospitals and Health Care in Brooklyn and New York, 1885–1915.* New York: Cambridge University Press, 1982.

Rothstein, William G. *American Medical Schools and the Practice of Medicine: A History.* New York: Oxford University Press, 1987.

Savacool, J. Woodrow. "Philadelphia and the White Plague," *Transactions and Studies of the College of Physicians of Philadelphia* 5th ser. 8 (1986): 147–181.

Scheffey, Lewis C. "The Early Years of the Obstetrical Society of Philadelphia." *Transactions and Studies of the College of Physicians of Philadelphia* 4th ser. 6 (1938/39): 125–147, 292–316.

Scranton, Philip, and Walter Licht. *Work Sights: Industrial Philadelphia, 1890–1950.* Philadelphia: Temple University Press, 1986.

Shafer, Henry Burnell, *The American Medical Profession, 1783 to 1850.* New York: Columbia University Press, 1936.

Shoemaker, Susan T. "The Philadelphia Pediatric Society and its Milk Commission, 1896–1917: An Aspect of Urban Progressive Reform." *Pennsylvania History* 53 (1986): 273–288.

Shortland, Michael. *Medicine and Film: A Checklist, Survey and Research Resource.* Research Publications Number IX. Oxford: Wellcome Unit for the History of Medicine, [1989].

Shryock, Richard. "The Advent of Modern Medicine in Philadelphia, 1800–1850." *Yale Journal of Biological Medicine* 13 (1940/41): 715–738.

————. "A Century of Medical Progress in Philadelphia, 1750–1850," *Pennsylvania History* 8 (1941): 7–28.

Smith, D. C. "The Emergence of Organized Clinical Instruction in the Nineteenth-Century American Cities of Boston, New York, and Philadelphia." Ph.D. dissertation, University of Minnesota, Minneapolis, 1979.

Solis-Cohen, Myer. "The Old Philadelphia Laryngological Society of the 1880s." *Annals of Medical History* 3rd ser. 3 (1941): 114–127.

Sontag, Susan. *On Photography.* New York: Farrar, Strauss & Giroux, 1977.

Spiller, W. G. "The First Fifty Years of the Philadelphia Neurological Society." *Archives of Neurology and Psychiatry* 34 (1935): 899–906.

Stachniewiecz, Stephanie A. and Jean K. Axelrod. *The Double Frill: The History of the Philadelphia General Hospital School of Nursing.* Philadelphia: Stickley, 1978.

Stapp, William F. *Robert Cornelius: Portraits from the Dawn of Photography.* Washington, D.C.: Smithsonian Institution Press for the National Portrait Gallery, 1983.

Starr, Paul. *The Social Transformation of American Medicine.* New York: Basic Books, 1982.

Stephenson, L. W. "Reflections on the Military Involvement of a Medical School." *Surgical Gynecology and Obstetrics* 154 (1982): 888–896.

Stevens, Rosemary. *American Medicine and the Public Interest.* New Haven, Conn.: Yale University Press, 1971.

———. *In Sickness and in Wealth: American Hospitals in the Twentieth Century.* New York: Basic Books, 1989.

———. "'A Poor Sort of Memory': Voluntary Hospitals and Government Before the Great Depression." *Health and Society* 60 (1982): 551–584.

———. "Sweet Charity: State Aid to Hospitals in Pennsylvania, 1870–1910." *Bulletin of the History of Medicine* 58 (1984): 287–314, 474–495.

Stoeckle, John D., and George Abbott White. *Plain Pictures of Plain Doctoring.* Cambridge, Mass.: MIT Press, 1985.

Stokes, William Standley, Jr. *A Legend of Service to Children,* New York: The Newcomen Society in North America, 1960.

Tasman, William. *The History of Wills Eye Hospital.* Hagerstown, Md.: Harper & Row, 1980.

Thomas, Alan. *Time in a Frame: Photography and the Nineteenth-Century Mind.* New York: Schocken, 1977.

Thompson, John D. and Grace Goldin. *The Hospital: A Social and Architectural History.* New Haven, Conn.: Yale University Press, 1975.

Thorpe, Francis Newton. *William Pepper, M.D., LL.D., 1843–1898.* Philadelphia: Lippincott, 1904.

Tomes, Nancy. *A Generous Confidence: Thomas Story Kirkbride and the Art of Asylum-Keeping, 1840–1883.* New York: Cambridge University Press, 1984.

———. "'Little World of Our Own': The Pennsylvania Hospital Training School for Nurses, 1895–1907." *Journal of the History of Medicine* 33 (1978): 507–533.

Trachtenberg, Alan. *Reading American Photographs: Images as History, Mathew Brady to Walker Evans*. New York: Hill & Wang, 1989.

VanderVeer, Joseph B. *Cardiology at the Pennsylvania Hospital, 1920–1980*. Bryn Mawr, Pa.: Published by the author, 1986.

Vogel, Morris J. *The Invention of the Modern Hospital, Boston, 1870–1930*. Chicago: University of Chicago Press, 1980.

———. "Machine Politics and Medical Care: The City Hospital at the Turn of the Century." In Charles E. Rosenberg, ed., *The Therapeutic Revolution: Essays in the Social History of American Medicine*, pp. 159–175. Philadelphia: University of Pennsylvania Press, 1979.

Wagner, Frederick B. *Thomas Jefferson University: Tradition and Heritage*. Philadelphia: Lea & Febiger, 1989.

Wagner, Jon, ed. *Images of Information: Still Photography in the Social Sciences*. Beverly Hills, Calif.: Sage, 1979.

Walsh, Mary Roth. *"Doctors Wanted, No Women Need Apply": Sexual Barriers in the Medical Profession, 1835–1975*. New Haven, Conn.: Yale University Press, 1977.

Ward, H. B. "Founder of American Parasitology, Joseph Leidy." *Journal of Parasitology* 10 (1924): 1–21.

Warner, John Harley. *The Therapeutic Perspective: Medical Practice, Knowledge, and Identity in America, 1820–1885*. Cambridge, Mass.: Harvard University Press, 1986.

Weigley, Russel F., ed. *Philadelphia: A 300-Year History*. New York: Norton, 1982.

Wessell, Henry W. *History of the Jewish Hospital Association of Philadelphia*. Philadelphia: Stern, 1908.

West, Roberta M. *History of Nursing in Pennsylvania*. Harrisburg, Pa.: Pennsylvania State Nurses' Association, 1939.

Whiteman, Maxwell. *Mankind and Medicine: A History of Philadelphia's Albert Einstein Medical Center*. Philadelphia: Albert Einstein Medical Center, 1966.

Williams, William H. *America's First Hospital: The Pennsylvania Hospital, 1751–1841*. Wayne, Pa.: Haverford House, 1976.

Wolf, Edwin, II. *Philadelphia, Portrait of an American City: A Bicentennial History*. Harrisburg, Pa.: Stackpole Books, 1975.

Index